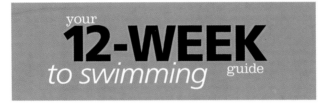

# your
# 12-WEEK
## *to swimming* guide

**FROM YOUR ARMCHAIR TO A 400-METRE SWIM IN 12 WEEKS**

Fact box sources (note: conversions are from g to oz (US) and from ml to fl oz (US). (1) UK Department of Health. (2) USGS. (3) UK Department of Health. (4) UK Department of Health: Sport and Exercise Medicine: a Fresh Approach (2012). (5) McDonald's, Pizza Hut, KFC (all US). (6) P Lally, European Journal of Social Psychology. (7) US National Health Interview Survey (2010). (8) Harvard Heart Letter (July 2004). (9) Coca-Cola (US), Starbucks (US). (10) UK Department of Health. Start Active, Stay Active (2011) and US The President's Council on Physical Fitness and Sport. (11) UK Department of Health: Start Active, Stay Active (2011) and www.bootsdiets.com. (12) US National Sleep Foundation. (13) UK NHS Sport and Exercise Medicine: A Fresh Approach (2011). (14) US The President's Council on Physical Fitness and Sports: Fast Facts About Sports Nutrition. (15) Drinkaware.co.uk. (16) US The President's Council on Physical Fitness and Sports: Fast Facts About Sports Nutrition. (17) US The President's Council on Physical Fitness and Sports: Exercise and Weight Control. (18) AM Williamson and AM Feyer, British Medical Journal (2000). (19) USGS. (20) Fitness Australia. (21) *Triathlon: Serious About Your Sport* (NHP). (22) Olaf Lahl et al, University of Dusseldorf (2008). (23) JH Stubbe et al, The association between exercise participation and well-being (2006) and various others. Photos: iStockphoto.com and www.sxu.hu, P19 Brandon W Mosley, www..manjidesigns.com. P20 Svilen Milev, www.effective.com. P30 Daino_16, http://leoele.blogspot.co.uk/search/label/photography. P36 Meral Akbulut. P39 Alx Sanchez, www.alxsanchex.com. P40 Scott Snyder, www.clearcaptures.com. P42 Marius Largu, www.lartekgrup.com. P49 Julia Reinikka, www.eggshell.com.au. P62 Luz Maria Espinoza, analab01. P64 PLRANG Images for design, www.phototric.com. P71 Manfred Werner. www.wikimedia.org. P72 Chris Coudron, http://chriscoudron.com. P74 Richard Dudley, www.bluegumgraphics.com.au. P77 Meral Akbulut. P81 Luz Maria Espinoza, analab01. P87 Tolga Kostak. P88 Chris Coudron, http://chriscoudron.com. P91 Alfredo Camacho, www.coroflot.com/alfredocb/trabalhos. P92 Meral Akbulut. P100 Charles Thompson, www.cameraclash.com. P104 snowee. P106 Graham Briggs, www.dreamstime.com/GBfoto_portfolio_pg1. P109 and P116 Janusz Gawron, www.januszgawron.pl. P114 Scott Snyder, www.clearcaptures.com. P120 Lisa Gaith. P124 Zsuzsanna Kilian. P126 Paulo Meira, www.unitdesign.com. P143 Craig Toron.

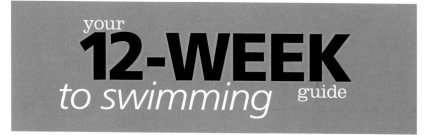

# your
# 12-WEEK
## *to swimming* guide

**FROM YOUR ARMCHAIR TO A 400-METRE SWIM IN 12 WEEKS**

by Daniel Ford

Training programme by Adam Dickson

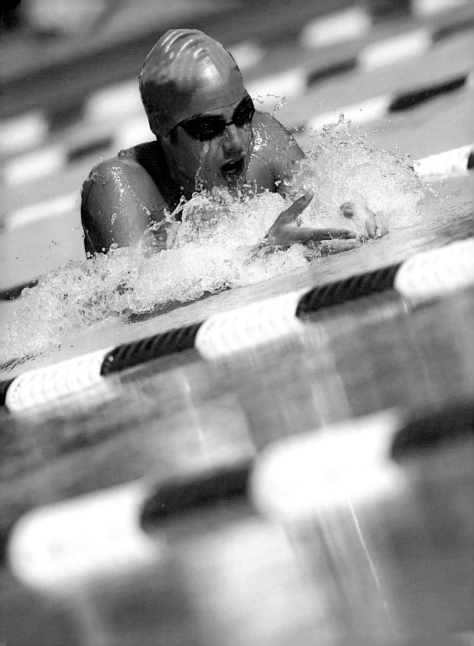

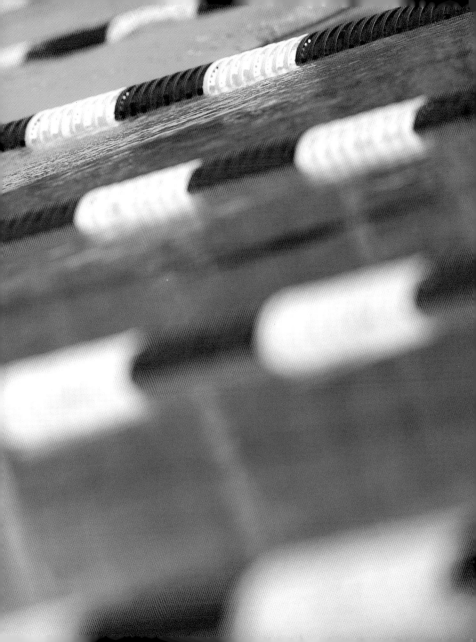

# your **12-WEEK** plan

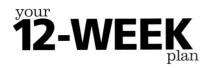

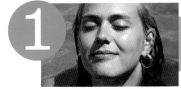

## Commit to the challenge

Tell other people what you intend to do…

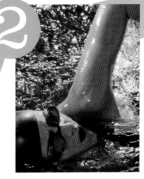

## Settling in

The programme is underway, so slowly and gently settle into your swimming…

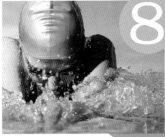

## Keep it going

Well done! You are heading into the second half of the the programme…

## Recommit to your swim

Look ahead to the finish and recommit to the 400-metre challenge…

## Taking care of details

It's time to refine your technique…

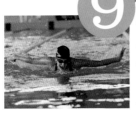

## Keep on track

You're feeling strong but don't get over-confident…

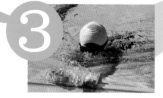

### 3

## Now stretch and relax

Stretching and resting are integral to your training programme…

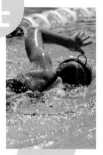

### 4

## Swimming can be a habit

Before you know it swimming will be a part of your routine…

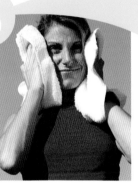

### 6

## Enjoy the benefits

You have been working hard, so now you can enjoy feeling fitter…

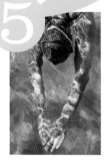

### 5

## Smooth rhythm

You should be feeling more comfortable in the pool now. Enjoy the rhythm of it…

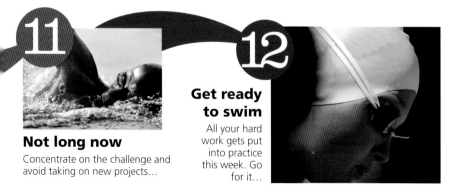

### 11

## Not long now

Concentrate on the challenge and avoid taking on new projects…

### 12

## Get ready to swim

All your hard work gets put into practice this week. Go for it…

# introduction

## Get ready to start your swimming challenge...

**Most of us** are very good at putting things off. Chances are you have been meaning to drag yourself from your armchair and start exercising for quite some time now. But somehow there is always a reason to put it off isn't there? Sometimes it's a work commitment, sometimes it's something at home that needs sorting out. "I'll just get this out the way then I'll make a start on my fitness," you might have promised yourself umpteen times before. Excuses, excuses, excuses.

The good news is you have broken that line of thought already, because the most important step in achieving anything new is simply deciding to do it. Once you have made the decision you set the ball rolling towards success. So you decided those double-cheese pizzas were no longer the way forward for you, went out and bought this book, and now the fitness ball is rolling. Granted, there is still 12 weeks of work ahead but the all-important first step has been taken. And there was you thinking the first step was the hardest.

Throughout this book you will see motivational quotes by people from different walks of life. You

# one

*There is only one thing you should be concentrating on right now and that is to start exercising. Don't attempt to give up smoking and drinking, and start eating salads just yet. You are more likely to give up if you try to change too much at once.*

"Success is not
for the timid. It
is for those who
seek guidance,
make decisions,
and take
decisive action."

**JOSE SILVA**

can draw on these to help you along the way – and even find your own favourites – but remember that at the end of the day you are the only one who can get yourself to the end goal of the 400-metre swim.

Don't look ahead and worry about the big 12-week chunk of exercise that has been set out before you. Instead, simply approach it as you would a large project at work. You don't panic about the delivery of the project, you simply set about breaking it down into small, manageable chunks. What needs doing and who are the best people in the office to do these things? How long will each element take? What do we need from outside and which suppliers are the best to deliver these? You are effectively piecing together a series of small parts to create the whole – the project. And so it is with this swimming challenge. By taking each session at a time, each week at a time, you are putting the fitness blocks together so you are ready for the 400-metre swim at the end.

An excellent exercise at this stage is to visualize your success. A lot of people dismiss this but remember your mind and body work together all the time. Top athletes spend a lot of time on visualization because they know how important it is. They will think through what they are going to do from start to finish and they will keep repeating it over and over again. Their minds are preparing their bodies for what lies ahead.

## hear

*Listen to your body. You know when you are feeling good and you know when you are not because your body tells you. Follow the programme and listen to advice but always remember the best guide you will have is your own body.*

# see

Take a few moments now to think through what is ahead of you. It's better to find somewhere quiet to do this and you might find it helps if you close your eyes. Remember, you are programming your mind so keep your thoughts positive. Picture yourself in your swimming kit on the day of the challenge, feeling strong and happy. You have just completed the 400-metre swim and you are looking forward to going into work so you can proudly tell your colleagues how well you did. This doesn't have to take more than a couple of minutes but by picturing your success you are setting your mind and your body on the path to completing this swimming challenge in 12 weeks.

## How to use your book

Right, now you've pictured the end result in your mind it's time to start taking the steps needed to get there. You won't need to be a rocket scientist to realize that this book is broken down into 12 large steps. Each will include a brief overview of what the focus of that particular week is all about. Read this at the end of the previous week so you've got time to digest it. As with above, visualize the success of the week (come on, you're an old hand at this). Don't skip these few seconds of visualization as they are important in firming up the week ahead in your mind. You will also find snippets of information on things such as food and drink, mental fitness, sleep, and so on that you can use during your 12 weeks.

The most important page in each section is Your Training Programme and Diary. Again, look over this page at the end of the previous week so the information has plenty of time to sink in. Also ensure you make space in your diary for each day's activity and don't relegate them to, "I'll fit that in somewhere," or you'll get to the end of the day and realize there is no time left. Treat each session as you would an important meeting at work or an appointment at your child's school.

At the bottom of these pages you will also see some traffic lights offering a 'Do This', 'Consider This' and a 'Don't Do This'. These are small tips that you can take on board during the week. You will also see a 'Reward' on this page, a little something to look forward to when the week is completed. Thoughtful eh? Ah, it's nothing. Use the small notes column to the right of each day to record how you're feeling. It's a great way to end a session and fun to look back on later. You will be amazed at how quickly you will progress.

Finally, at the end of each chapter there is a summary of what you have achieved that week. Again, use the notes column to jot down your thoughts and feelings as this will draw a line under the week and help prepare you for the next one. Then it's time for you to give yourself a pat on the back and refer back to your reward.

when

*When thinking of taking up an exercise programme for the first time or after an extended break it's important that you check with your doctor that you are fit and healthy enough. Explain your plan and get the thumbs up before starting.*

## Your aim this week

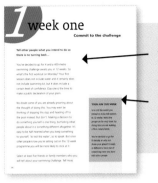

At the end of each week read what's in store for the coming week so you have time to digest it.

This is where you will find a snapshot of your aim for the week. Elsewhere in the section you will find small snippets of information on things such as food and drink or mental fitness.

## Training programme

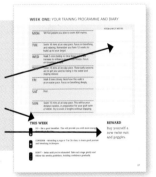

Make sure you diarize your sessions as if they are important appointments. They are.

Jot down your thoughts even if it's just, "Saw Mrs Smith as I set off for the pool. She looked impressed!" or "Felt great today".

These are additional tips you can use during your week.

This is what you are looking forward to at the end of the week.

## What you have achieved

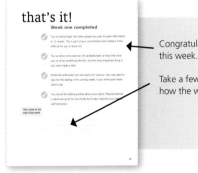

Congratulations, this is what you have completed this week.

Take a few moments to jot down your thoughts on how the week went, whether it was good or bad.

# *1* week one

## Commit to the challenge

**Tell other people what you intend to do so there is no turning back…**

You've decided to go for it and a 400-metre swimming challenge awaits you in 12 weeks. So what's the first workout on Monday? Your first session does not include water and it certainly does not include swimming kit, but it does include a certain level of confidence. Day one is the time to make a public declaration of your plans.

No doubt some of you are already groaning about the thought of doing this. You may even be thinking of skipping this step and heading off to the pool instead. But don't. Making a decision to do something yourself is one thing, but telling other people about it is something different altogether. It's easy to be half-hearted when you keep something to yourself, 'to test the water', so to speak. But once other people know you're setting out on this 12-week programme you will be more likely to stick at it.

Select at least five friends or family members who you will tell about your swimming challenge. Tell more

### YOUR AIM THIS WEEK

Is to tell the world you intend to swim 400 metres in 12 weeks. Well, five people at the very least. By doing this you are making a firm commitment.

You've decided to go for it already so why not share your plans? It really is difficult to back out of something once you have told other people.

"The achievement of your goal is assured the moment you commit yourself to it."

**MACK R DOUGLAS**

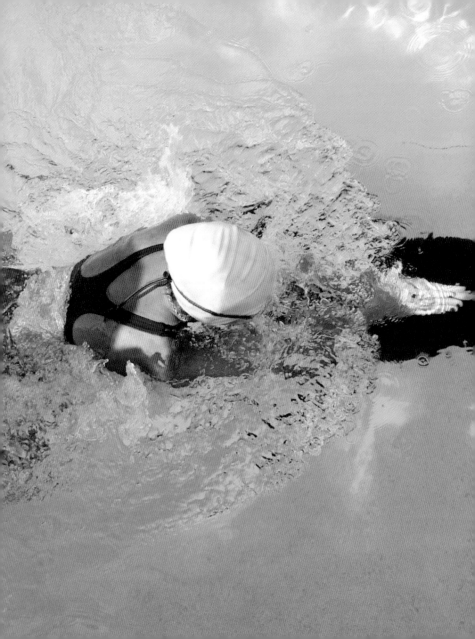

# **WEEK ONE:** YOUR TRAINING PROGRAMME AND DIARY

| | | YOUR DAILY NOTES |
|---|---|---|
| **MON** | Tell five people you plan to swim 400 metres. | |
| **TUE** | Swim 10 mins at an easy pace. Focus on breathing and relaxing. Remember you have 12 weeks to build up to your target. | |
| **WED** | Walk 5 mins briskly. In time these walks will increase to enhance your overall fitness. Focus on breathing deeply. | |
| **THU** | Swim 10 mins at an easy pace. These early sessions are to get you used to being in the water and staying relaxed. | |
| **FRI** | Walk 8 mins slowly. Note how this walk is at an easier pace. Focus on breathing deeply. | |
| **SAT** | Rest. | |
| **SUN** | Swim 15 mins at an easy pace. This is your distance session. Try to swim 50 metres (2 lengths) without stopping. | |

## THIS WEEK

DO – Wear a swimming cap. As well as keeping your hair out of your eyes, it is likely to be compulsory in many swimming pools.

CONSIDER – Attending a yoga or T'ai Chi class, to learn good posture and breathing techniques.

DON'T – Swim until you're exhausted. Take each stage gently and follow the weekly guidelines, building confidence gradually.

## REWARD

**Buy yourself a new swim suit and goggles.**

people if you want to and by all means use social media to spread the word far and wide if you are feeling particularly confident. But don't hide behind your Twitter or Facebook announcements, as it's an important part of the process for you to tell some people face-to-face.

Don't go bouncing into work with your new fitness kit when you do this, no one likes a bore. You really do need people encouraging you at this stage so just keep it casual. When someone asks you what you did on the weekend you can proudly announce you bought a new book (feel free to point to it on your desk!) and have decided to follow the fitness programme.

Most people will be supportive but don't get put off if some are apathetic or even dismissive of your plans. Use any negative looks or comments to spur you on; proving people like this wrong can act as a motivator. But you really do need a few cheery pats on the back so make sure you tell a couple of people you know will support your plans (best friends and mums are good for this).

So that's it for day one. The rest of the week includes three short sessions in the water plus a couple of walks to keep you loose. The walks are important and will continue to be included in the programme for the coming weeks. Swimming is one of the toughest

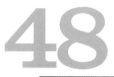

**48**

*Is the number of minutes you will be exercising this week. This is probably less than the time you might spend having a coffee with a friend or even watching your favourite television programme. Not a lot when you think of it like that is it? Make sure you find the time for exercise just as you would any other activity.*

"There are only two options regarding commitment. You're either in or out."

**PAT RILEY**

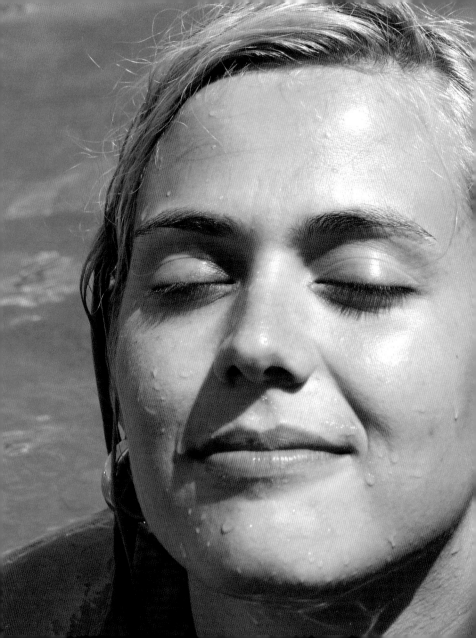

sports there is as you need to work your whole body as you push against the resistance of the water. The walks give you a break from this tough work while still contributing towards building your overall fitness.

As you have probably been out of the pool for a long time, take things easy. Concentrate getting into a steady breathing pattern and building a smooth stroke in these earlier sessions. Sundays will be when you do your 'long' swim. This week it is two lengths (assuming a standard 25m pool) and this target will increase gradually as you get fitter. However, remember these are still *targets* and you shouldn't worry if you can't complete what is set out in the programme. So don't be afraid to take a breather during these two lengths this week if you feel you need to.

The best thing about being at the start of something new is that mixture of excitement and apprehension you feel. It's not unlike being at an airport, passport and ticket in hand, as you check the boards for your flight to be called. Enjoy this feeling and tuck it away into your memory bank (plus write down how you feel in the notes' section provided). There will come times in the next few weeks when your enthusiasm is not as high. When these times do come, dig into your memory and draw on the feeling of excitement you are feeling now (plus re-read your notes). But for now enjoy that airport moment. Your flight has been called!

## Women doing enough exercise

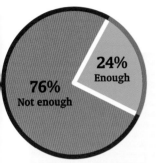

24%
Enough

76%
Not enough

Only 24 per cent of women (37 per cent of men) in the UK do enough exercise according to government health guidelines. Well done, you are on your way to joining the minority!

The figures show just how easy it is for most people to fall into the trap of not keeping fit. Remind yourself of this if you ever feel like giving up in the coming weeks. (1)

"Everything you can imagine is real."

**PABLO PICASSO**

# that's it!

## Week one completed

 You've told at least five other people you plan to swim 400 metres in 12 weeks. This is part of your commitment and makes it more difficult for you to back out.

 You've done some exercise. It's probably been a long time since you've done something like this, but the most important thing is you have made a start.

 Bottle the enthusiasm you are feeling for exercise. You may need to tap into this feeling in the coming weeks if your enthusiasm levels start to dip.

 You should be feeling positive about your plans. Physical exercise is obviously good for your body but it also improves your mental well-being too.

**Your notes at the end of the week**

# week two

## Settling into your swimming

**The programme is underway, so slowly and gently ease into your swimming...**

The early stages of this 12-week programme have been all about getting your mind right and committing yourself to completing this swimming challenge. You've also had a couple of gentle sessions in the pool and a couple of walks, but these were aimed at getting you used to being back in the water and exercising again.

Now is the time to really settle into your swimming. At the start of this week we recommend you book a session with a qualified swimming instructor so you can work on your technique and breathing. Instructors are not just for children learning to swim or top swimmers chasing an Olympic medal. Explain what you are doing and the programme you are following. Because you have been away from the pool for quite a while it will not be surprising if your technique is a bit rusty. And with that comes a lack of confidence, which can affect your breathing pattern. To get the most from this programme you need to have a smooth stroke and breathing pattern

### YOUR AIM THIS WEEK

Is to have a lesson with a swimming instructor. Explain what you are doing and ask for help with improving your technique and breathing.

Put the lessons you learn from the instructor into practice during the two other sessions in the water this week.

"A promise is a cloud; fulfilment is rain."

**ARABIAN PROVERB**

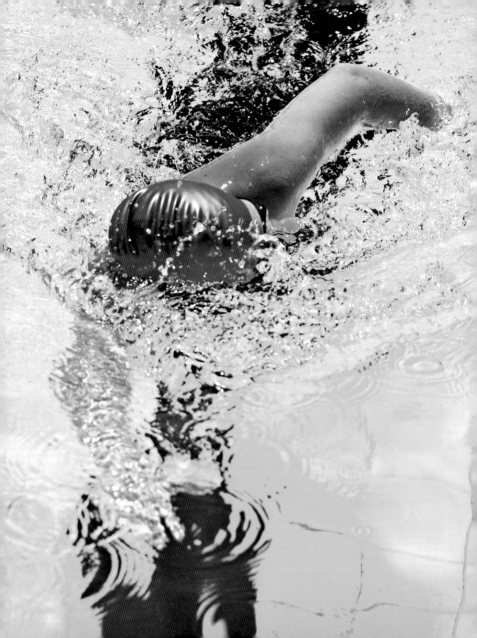

# WEEK TWO: YOUR TRAINING PROGRAMME AND DIARY

| | | |
|---|---|---|
| **MON** | Rest. Go about your daily routine and think about your goals. | |
| **TUE** | Swimming lesson with a qualified instructor. Here you can learn the technique and breathing that will help you towards your goal. | |
| **WED** | Walk 5 mins briskly. If you have learnt to breathe correctly, now is the time to put it into practice. | |
| **THU** | Swim 10 mins. Practise the technique and drills you have learned from your instructor. | |
| **FRI** | Walk 8 minutes slowly. | |
| **SAT** | Rest. | |
| **SUN** | Warm-up, then try to swim for 75 metres (3 lengths) without stopping. Rest for 5 mins, then cool down. Relax and focus on your breathing. | |

## THIS WEEK

DO – Practise the drills and technique taught by your swimming instructor as these will enhance your performance and save you valuable energy in the long run.

CONSIDER – Eating more complex carbohydrates, such as oats, pasta, vegetables and fruit and cut back on saturated fats, chocolate, pastries etc.

DON'T – Forget to warm-up and cool down. A few minutes gentle swimming before and after your main set will be ample.

## REWARD

Lie-in on Sunday morning – if you don't have small children!

as you swim, and a qualified instructor can help with this. There are a few recommended sessions with a swimming instructor in the programme, so this is a good opportunity to build a relationship with someone who can really help you as you train for your challenge.

Use the swims planned for the rest of the week to put the lessons you learn from your instructor, in particular your breathing, into practice. Remember Sunday is set aside for your long swim – this week the target increases by one length to three. But as mentioned previously, this is just a *target*, so do not worry if you can't manage it yet and you need to take a break.

Now you are back in the water it is important to take things steady. Time has moved on, so don't dive in and go thrashing around straight away as if you are still a teenager with boundless energy. What you can take from those years is the idea that being in the water is 'fun', so enjoy your swims as welcome breaks from your daily responsibilities. Swimming is an excellent way to exercise because it is non weight bearing, so it is ideal for people who can't run or do other types of exercise. It will also help tone your muscles and improve your posture.

Enjoy your time in the water and congratulate yourself that you are exercising again. But even if you

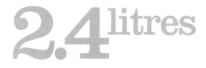

*Every day you need to replace 2.4 litres (five pints) of water that is lost or expelled from your body. Although some will come from the food you eat it's important that you drink plenty of water during the day to ensure you do not become dehydrated. (2)*

"No river can return to its source, yet all rivers must have a beginning."

**NATIVE AMERICAN PROVERB**

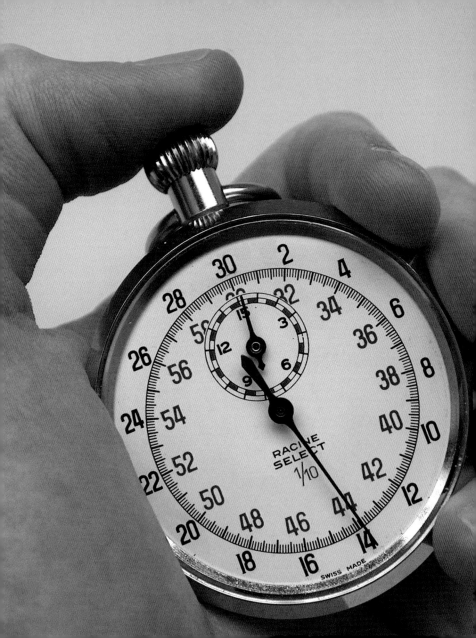

## Daily calorie intake

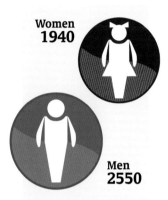

**Women**
**1940**

**Men**
**2550**

There is no need to get calorie obsessed but nutritional values are clearly marked on most food we buy so it's easy enough to keep an eye on your intake.

What you need per day depends on various factors such as your height, weight and your lifestyle. The chart shows the estimated averages by UK authorities. (3)

are feeling on top of the world at the moment, avoid the temptation to swim for longer than is set out in the programme or to go for an extra swim on a rest day. Doing too much at the start of a programme is common, but it's better to run the race like the tortoise and get where you want, than be like the hare and be nowhere to be seen at the end. Of course, you are the only one who truly knows how much you can do, but the programme is geared towards getting you to the 400-metre goal with a sure and steady progression, so stick to it.

Always listen to your body. If at any time you feel you have done too much during a session, stop and take a break, and if necessary cut the session short. If you feel exhausted during the week (not just the expected tiredness from exercising) then have an extra rest day. Do not push yourself beyond what your body is telling you it can manage.

One problem when you start exercising again after a break, is being self-conscious of your body. Thoughts like, "Do I look silly when I swim?" and "Does my excess weight show in this costume?" are common early on. Try not to care what other people think (most are usually more concerned with themselves anyway) as this challenge is all about you. However, if it really does concern you then you will need to find a quiet time at the pool (perhaps just as they open?) so you feel more comfortable.

"If you want to
do something,
do it!"
**PLAUTUS**

# that's it!

## Week two completed

 You have had a session with a swimming instructor to help you improve your technique and breathing. Concentrate on putting the lessons you learnt into practice every time you swim.

 You know you should stick to the programme, even if you are feeling super enthusiastic at the moment.

 You know you need to take things steady in these early swimming sessions. There is still plenty of time to get fit and complete this challenge successfully.

 You know that if you are feeling self-conscious about exercising you should find a time when the pool is quiet. Don't let a thing like this stop you.

Your notes at the
end of the week

# 3 week three

## Now stretch and relax

**Stretching and resting are integral to your training programme…**

Hands up who likes stress? Come on, don't all rush at once. Granted, the type of stress that comes from too many hours and ridiculous demands at work, is not good and nobody enjoys that. However, stress of a different kind is an integral part of your training. To build your strength and your cardiovascular fitness you need to put your body under a certain amount of stress. If you never push your muscles more than they are used to (ie. put them under stress) then they will never get stronger. And the same goes for your cardiovascular system. Now, let's try again. Hands up who likes stress?

But it's not as simple as that. You can't just keep stressing your body endlessly and keep reaping the rewards – you will just push it over the edge. To build strength and fitness – now here comes the good bit – you need plenty of rest too. After stressing your body (in the good way) with exercise, it needs to recover and rebuild itself. If it doesn't get the necessary recovery time then it won't be ready

**YOUR AIM THIS WEEK**

Is to treat your rest days with respect. These days are an integral part of the programme, as this is when your body recovers from the hard work it has done in the training sessions.

You should also be concentrating on getting into a good sleep pattern, and avoiding the habit of 'catching up' on weekends.

"The main thing
to do is relax and
let your talent do
the work."

**CHARLES BARKLEY**

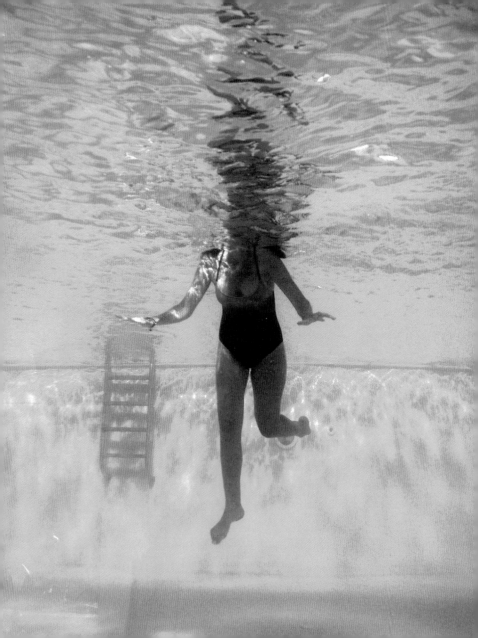

# WEEK THREE: YOUR TRAINING PROGRAMME AND DIARY

| | |
|---|---|
| **MON** | Rest. This week sees a slight reduction in the time you spend exercising, in order to prepare you for the next phase. |
| **TUE** | Warm-up, then try to swim 2 lengths. Rest for 30 seconds. Focus on technique and breathing. Repeat x 3. |
| **WED** | Walk 5 minutes briskly. |
| **THU** | Repeat Tuesday's set, focusing on technique and breathing. |
| **FRI** | Walk 5 mins slowly. Make this an extra session in addition to what you do in your daily life (such as walking to the bus stop). |
| **SAT** | Rest. |
| **SUN** | Warm-up, then swim 100 metres (4 lengths). Rest for 5 minutes, then cool down. Focus on relaxing and breathing. |

## THIS WEEK

 DO – Congratulate yourself on getting this far. By following the programme, you are one step nearer completion of your goal.

CONSIDER – Finding ways to relax when you are out of the pool. Read a book. Take a hot bath. Have a massage.

 DON'T – Compare yourself to other swimmers. Remind yourself that this is all about your own enjoyment and that the benefits are yours alone.

## REWARD

**Turn off your phone for an hour, put your feet up and relax.**

for the next session. That's why there are plenty of rest days built into the programme. Enjoy them in the knowledge that they are just as important as your training sessions.

Now 'rest' in reality, of course, is unlikely to mean doing absolutely nothing all day. After all, there are few of us who don't have work and family responsibilities to deal with. But try to set aside some time for relaxation during the day, whether it is enjoying a hot bath, watching a film or reading a book. Taking time like this means you will return to training feeling refreshed and raring to go.

So now on to sleep, the best rest you can get. Exercising regularly does, in general, help you sleep better. However, avoid scheduling your workout too close to your bedtime, as this will make it difficult for you to get to sleep. Also avoid taking stimulants such as alcohol, caffeine and nicotine too close to your bedtime for the same reason. Remember there is caffeine in chocolate, tea, soft drinks and some pain relievers, as well as coffee. Alcohol can make it easier to get to sleep but the quality of sleep you get after drinking will be poor.

You will get the best benefit from sleep if you get into a regular pattern so you are going to bed at the same time every night and waking at the same every morning. Of course, the reality of our modern,

# 38%

*Unless you're a particular fan of hospital food, being inactive doesn't really hold much appeal. UK research has found that inactive people spend 38 per cent more days in hospital than active people, visit their doctor 5.5 per cent more and use specialist services 13 per cent more.* (4)

"Movement is a medicine for creating change in a person's physical, emotional, and mental states."

**CAROL WELCH**

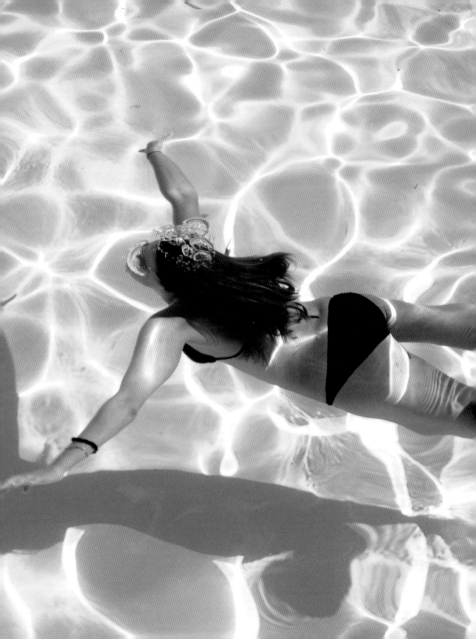

busy world, is that most of us spend the weekends 'catching up'. However, your body reacts badly to this as it disrupts your sleep cycle, so work hard at establishing a regular sleep pattern if you can.

Stretching is important for all athletes but it is especially important when you are swimming, because this is a sport where you are working all your muscles during your training sessions. Make sure you spend a few minutes stretching before every workout, being careful to do this very gently at the start, as your muscles will not be warm and supple at this point. Work methodically through each part of your body – the back of your legs (calves, hamstrings, glutes), the front of your legs (quads), your back, shoulders and neck, so you are loose and tension-free before your swim. Repeat the process at the end of your session as well, to avoid your muscles tightening up. Assuming you have been swimming in a nice, temperature-controlled pool, your muscles will be warm and receptive to being stretched.

You should consider stretching as an integral part of each training session (in fact, stretching is the one thing we would encourage you to do on your rest days), and not something to be fitted in only 'if time allows'. Some people view stretching as the 'soft' part of training but you will soon start to feel the benefits from just a few minutes working your muscles.

## Calories in takeaways

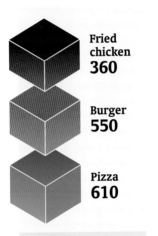

**Fried chicken**
**360**

**Burger**
**550**

**Pizza**
**610**

Nothing beats a tasty takeaway, but keep an eye on the calories. The chart above refers to a Big Mac (215 g, 7.6 oz), a Pizza Hut Pepperoni 6-inch (15 cm) Personal Pan Pizza, a KFC chicken breast (163 g, 5.8 oz). (5)

"A coach can inspire athletes, Motivation comes from within."

**ANON**

# that's it!

## Week three completed

 You recognize you need to stress your body to build your strength and cardiovascular fitness. Rest days are important to allow your body to recover.

 You know sleep is the best rest you can get. Get into a regular sleep pattern so you are going to bed at the same time every night and waking at the same time every morning.

 You always spend a few minutes stretching out your muscles, both before and after a training session.

 You will aim to do some stretching on your rest days to help keep you loose for the next session.

Your notes at the end of the week

# week four

## Swimming can become a habit

**Before you know it swimming will be a part of your routine…**

Good habits are wonderful things because you don't even need to think about doing them, they just happen naturally. It's simple enough to form a habit: you keep repeating the same action over and over, until it is engrained and it will become a habit – it's as simple as that. The good news is that once a habit is formed it's pretty tough to break.

By following this programme towards the 400-metre swim challenge you have started sowing the seeds for a good habit. Keep working hard and the more time passes, the more engrained the action of training will become. Then, before you know it you'll be heading off to the pool with your kit packed without even thinking about it. Bingo! The habit is formed.

It's early days, so training will still be fresh and exciting, but it's unlikely it's a part of your routine just yet. So how long does it take? The time it takes for a habit to become engrained will vary from

**YOUR AIM THIS WEEK**

Is to keep working hard until exercise becomes a habit in your life.

If you keep repeating the same action often enough it becomes a habit – it's as simple as that. Soon you will be packing up your training kit and heading off to the swimming pool without even thinking about it.

"The habit
must become
easy. The easy
must become
beautiful."

**DOUG HENNING**

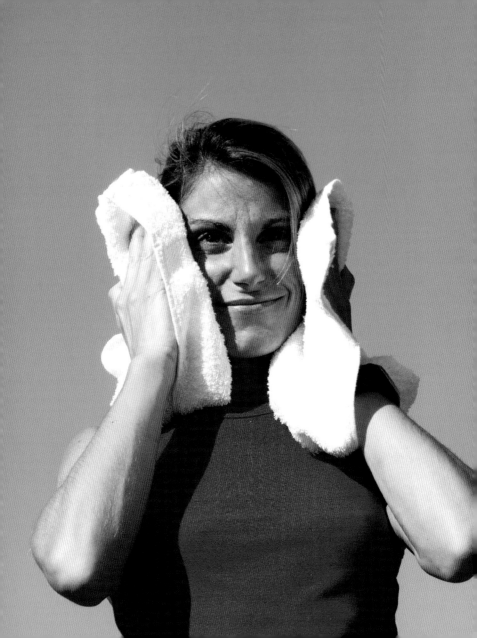

# WEEK FOUR: YOUR TRAINING PROGRAMME AND DIARY

| | |
|---|---|
| **MON** | Rest. This week sees an increase in the overall time spent exercising. Keep your goal in mind and take it easy. |
| **TUE** | Swimming lesson with a qualified instructor. Take note of any errors in your technique since the last lesson and aim to put them right. |
| **WED** | Walk 8 mins briskly. |
| **THU** | Warm-up, then swim 50 metres (2 lengths). Rest for 20 secs. Focus on technique and breathing. Repeat x 3. |
| **FRI** | Walk 10 minutes slowly. |
| **SAT** | Rest. |
| **SUN** | Warm-up, then swim 100 metres (4 lengths). Rest for 5 mins, then cool down. This distance swim will increase in the coming weeks. |

## THIS WEEK

DO – Make any changes suggested by your swimming instructor. Remember that good technique will improve your overall performance.

CONSIDER – Varying the speed of your sets. Try alternating two lengths moderate with two easy, remembering to rest adequately in-between.

DON'T – Force yourself to complete a session if you have a cold or feel ill. Apart from the fact that you could endanger your health, from a fitness perspective there is nothing to be gained.

## REWARD

Treat yourself to a professional massage.

person to person so stick to the programme and keep going.

Think of it this way: you didn't make a conscious decision to get out of shape as you became the pizza shop's favourite customer did you? No shame in that, the pressures of life – work, family and so on – simply crept up on you and before you knew it, eating a takeaway in your armchair while watching TV was the norm every night. You did it regularly and it became a habit. But now you are exercising regularly (and unlike the above, you *did* make a conscious decision to do it) and this in due course will become a habit.

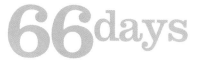

> *It takes an average of 66 days to form a habit. Although this is the average time it takes to turn something new into automatic behaviour a habit can form quicker for some or take considerably longer for others – so stick at it and exercise will soon become a habit for you.* (6)

There are a few things you can do to help this process to get engrained. You are already scheduling your training sessions into your diary as we suggested aren't you? Keep doing that and take a bit of time to look ahead so you can fill up your diary with all the sessions set out in the training programme. Yes, yes, we know you don't like planning ahead, but if you put in all the sessions as if they are important appointments, then you are unlikely to book something else that clashes with a training session.

You should also consider teaming up with a training buddy (if you haven't already done so). There are many benefits of training with someone else. You will both be able to encourage each other when the

"He who stops getting better stops being good."

**OLIVER CROMWELL**

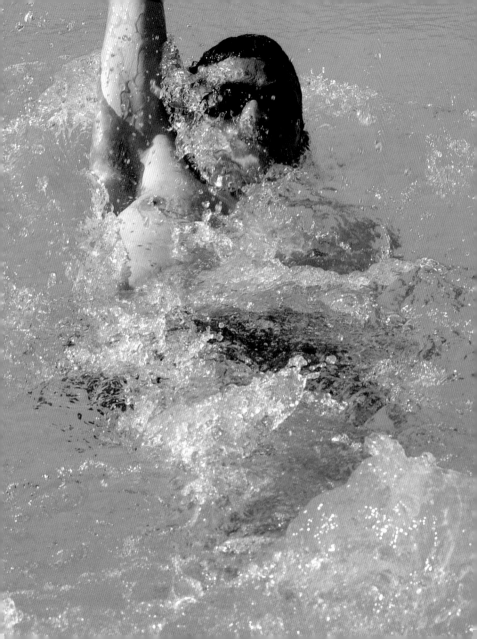

## How many people get enough sleep?

**70%**
**Enough sleep**

**30%**
**Not enough sleep**

Thirty per cent of working adults do not sleep enough (defined as less than six hours on average per day) according to a US survey.

A lack of sleep is associated with various health problems and makes it particularly difficult to train hard and get fit so make sure your lifestyle allows you to be part of the 70 per cent. (7)

going gets tough, and there are always times when a friendly word will help keep you going. You can reciprocate when you are feeling on top of the world and your buddy is struggling. But the best thing of having a training buddy is that it is very difficult to skip a session, or worse, give up altogether. You made a commitment to five people at the start of this programme in part to make it difficult to back out. If you start training with someone then that commitment becomes even stronger. It really is difficult to turn over in bed for an extra half hour's sleep when you know your training partner is waiting for you at the swimming pool.

Try to find someone who is more or less at the same fitness level as you, as you want to be able to work together. You don't want to be struggling to keep up with your buddy or vice versa.

You should also make sure you schedule your training sessions at a time when you won't be disrupted. Don't aim for swims if you have a family to get ready for school, and avoid after-work plans if you know your boss expects you to stay late sometimes. But maybe there is a pool near work and lunchtimes are a good time? Of course, you can't control everything, and there will also be time when there are commitments that have to override even your best-laid plans. However, by thinking ahead and choosing a time that suits you, the chances of this happening are reduced.

"Divide each difficulty into as many parts as necessary to resolve it."

**DESCARTES**

# that's it!

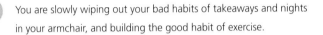

## Week four completed

 You are slowly wiping out your bad habits of takeaways and nights in your armchair, and building the good habit of exercise.

 You know it takes time to build good habits, so you need to keep working hard at this programme and soon the exercise habit will have taken root.

 You are treating every training session as you would any other important appointment so you will not miss them easily. Schedule them into your diary to help with this.

 You have found a time in the day that means you can train without disruption. Avoid times when you know you are usually busy with other commitments.

Your notes at the
end of the week

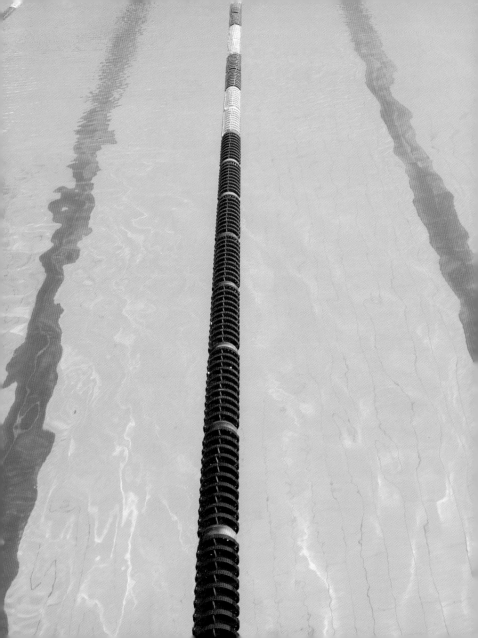

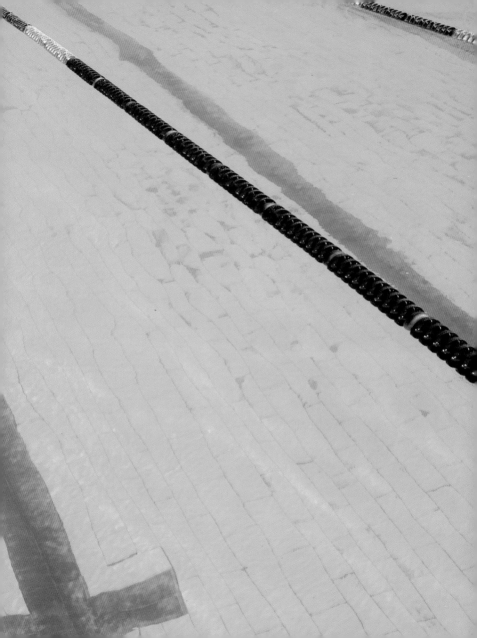

# week five

## The smooth rhythm of swimming

**You should be feeling more comfortable in the pool now. Enjoy the rhythm of swimming...**

When you return to the swimming pool after an extended break (how long was it?) you often feel a bit awkward. Sure, it's unlikely you had forgotten how to swim in the sense that you sunk to the bottom of the pool. But it is likely you forgot to swim in that nice, smooth rhythm that has you cutting through the water with ease.

Granted, you might not be leaping along like a youthful dolphin just yet, but a bit of that original pool rustiness should have disappeared from your body. It doesn't take long for your muscles to remember the most efficient way of operating so, although we are only a few weeks into the programme, you will already be starting to feel more comfortable in the water. Can there be a better feeling than the one of gliding gracefully along as if no effort is needed at all?

The best way to improve at swimming is to swim, swim, and swim some more, so in the coming weeks

### YOUR AIM THIS WEEK

Is to spend a bit of time looking at your swimming technique.

There is no need to become a technical swimming guru, because your body is good at adapting on its own. However, take a few minutes to think through your stroke to ensure it is smooth.

"All rewards
come from doing
not knowing."

**ANON**

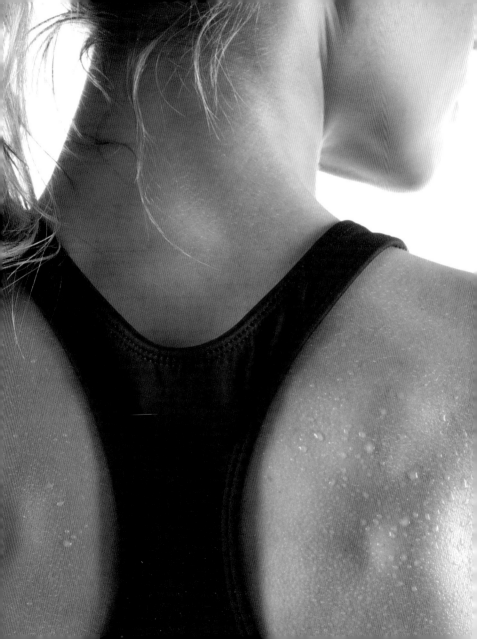

# WEEK FIVE: YOUR TRAINING PROGRAMME AND DIARY

| | | YOUR DAILY NOTES |
|---|---|---|
| **MON** | Rest. Try to visualize your form in the water, particularly how you use your hands. Practise this standing up in front of a mirror. | |
| **TUE** | Warm-up, then swim 75 metres (3 lengths). Rest for 20 seconds. Focus on technique and breathing. Repeat x 2. | |
| **WED** | Walk 8 mins briskly. | |
| **THU** | Warm-up, then swim 50 metres (2 lengths). Rest for 20 seconds. Focus on technique and breathing. Repeat x 4. | |
| **FRI** | Walk 10 minutes slowly. | |
| **SAT** | Rest. | |
| **SUN** | Warm-up, then swim 150 metres (6 lengths). Rest for 5 minutes, then cool down. Focus on an easy stroke and comfortable breathing. | |

## THIS WEEK

 DO – Aim to get more sleep as the sessions increase. Get to bed earlier rather than lie-in later in the morning. Sleep enhances all stages of growth and will improve your overall fitness.

 CONSIDER – Drinking more water throughout the day. Aim for a glass after each meal to re-hydrate and aid digestion. Also take a drinks bottle for before and after your swim.

DON'T – Give up! You're almost at the halfway stage. Results come from consistency and regular effort. The long-term health benefits are well worth the effort.

## REWARD

**Buy yourself some relaxing bath salts and enjoy a long, hot soak.**

you are going to continue to feel improvements in your style as well as your fitness. Your body is remarkably clever at finding the best way of doing something, so at this early stage try to relax during your swims and trust it. However, you can help things along nicely by taking a bit of time to look at your swimming technique.

Don't worry, we are not expecting you to become a technical guru overnight. Concentrating too much on every tiny little element of your stroke right now could distract you from the overall aim of getting fit enough for your 400-metre swim. However, take a bit of time to think through your stroke to ensure it is smooth. A jarring stroke will take more effort out of you.

That is why we recommend you take a bit of time on your rest day on Monday to visualize (that word again!) your stroke. Once you've run through the stroke in your head, stand in front of a mirror and practise your stroke through the air, paying particular attention to the shape of your hands. Again, this might seem strange to some people, but can it really be more strange than playing air guitar, which just about *everyone* has done at some stage!

Remember that when you are swimming, unlike most other sports, you will be using virtually every muscle group at the same time. Whatever stroke you prefer

## 30mins

*When running at a pace of 8 kph (5 mph) for 30 minutes a person weighing 56 kg (125 pounds) will burn 240 calories, while for someone weighing 70 kg (155 pounds) it is 298 calories, and at 84 kg (185 pounds) it is 355 calories. Figures are the same for circuit training, while swimming breaststroke burns 300, 372 and 444 calories respectively. For cycling at 19-22 kph (12-14 mph) the calories burnt are 240, 298 and 355. (8)*

"If it's not fun you're not doing it right."

**FRAN TARKETON**

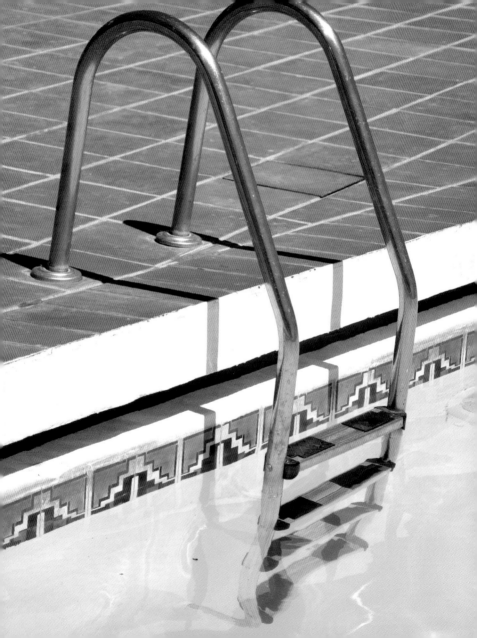

## Calories in drinks

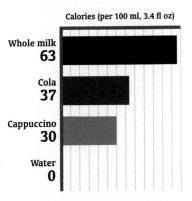

Calories (per 100 ml, 3.4 fl oz)

Whole milk
**63**

Cola
**37**

Cappuccino
**30**

Water
**0**

It's easy to rack up the calories you consume in drinks each day. Don't cut back and become dehydrated, just balance the type of drinks you enjoy. The chart shows figures for a glass of milk, Coca-Cola and a Starbucks cappuccino with whole milk. (9)

to use – we would advise breaststroke at this stage – the principles for making the stroke more efficient are the same. Although you will have your favourite stroke don't be afraid to experiment with the others (although maybe not too much butterfly which really is tough!). This will not only maintain your interest in swimming but will also strengthen muscles that in turn will help improve your preferred stroke.

To get the maximum from each stroke, concentrate on using your arms and legs in unison, getting the best 'kick' and 'pull' from your feet and hands respectively, and try to maintain a nice streamlined position in the water so as to reduce the resistance of your body in the water. Breathing is particularly important when swimming and is easy to get wrong because it's not something we normally have to think about. Concentrate on keeping your breathing pattern smooth and avoid gasping for breath on every stroke, as this will interrupt your stroke and increase your chance of getting a mouthful of water.

Have you bought yourself some proper swimming kit, hat and goggles yet? You can swim in a baggy pair of shorts or an ill-fitting costume if you want to, but built-for-purpose swimming kit, made of modern fabrics, is certainly better. Good swimwear is designed to reduce 'drag' in water, whereas beachwear will absorb more water and will make it harder for you to move through the water smoothly.

"If we are ever to enjoy life, now is the time, not tomorrow or next year... Today should always be our most wonderful day."

**THOMAS DREIER**

# that's it!

## Week five completed

 You are now enjoying the rhythm of swimming.

 You know the best way to improve is to swim, swim, and swim some more.

 You have taken a bit of time to think about your technique, in particular the shape of your hands. Improving your technique will improve your performance in the water.

 You should have bought some decent swimming kit, a hat and goggles. Getting some nice kit shows you are taking this seriously and will make you feel more positive.

Your notes at the
end of the week

# week six

## Enjoy the benefits of feeling fit

**You've been working hard, so you can now enjoy feeling fitter…**

The joys of feeling fit and healthy really are hard to beat. Sleeping better, then waking up feeling refreshed and raring to go (even if you are a little stiff), is a great feeling. The day feels like it is there to be enjoyed, and hey, you even have a spring in your step in the afternoons while others in the office are starting to wilt.

We don't need to preach about the well-known health benefits of exercise (good for your heart, helps you fight disease, and so on), but the changes you made a few weeks ago are already translating into making you a healthier person. Good for you, enjoy it. Even just a few weeks into the programme you should already be feeling more energetic (it's good for your sex life, too, by the way), but the benefits also extend to your mind.

Exercising really does improve your mood. The positive feeling you have right at the end of a swim starts to extend itself the more you make exercise a

**YOUR AIM THIS WEEK**

Is to enjoy all the benefits of feeling fitter and healthier.

Whether it is sleeping better, a renewed energy in the day, or feeling more positive, these are your benefits to enjoy after all your hard work. Remember that regular exercising has mental as well as physical benefits.

"May you live
all the days
of your life."

**JONATHAN SWIFT**

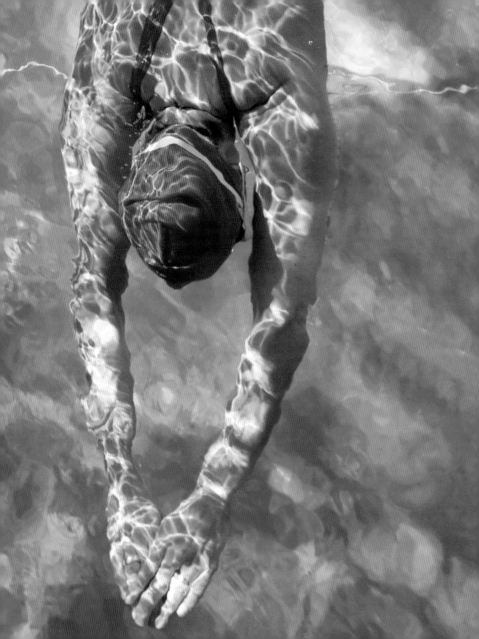

YOUR DAILY NOTES

| | | |
|---|---|---|
| **MON** | Rest. You're approaching the midway point so re-evaluate your goals. What improvements have you made? Which areas could you improve? | |
| **TUE** | Swimming lesson with qualified instructor. Make sure you ask if there's anything you're not sure about. | |
| **WED** | Walk 5 mins briskly. | |
| **THU** | Warm-up, thenswim 25 metres (1 length). Rest for 15 secs. Focus on technique and breathing. Repeat x 8. | |
| **FRI** | Walk 8 mins slowly. | |
| **SAT** | Rest. | |
| **SUN** | Warm-up, then swim 100 metres (4 lengths). Rest for 5 mins, then cool down. Focus on a relaxed stroke and good breathing. | |

## THIS WEEK

DO – Ensure you stick to the plan during the rest days. The reduced exercise allows the mind and body to recuperate, preparing you for the next phase.

CONSIDER – Reviewing your technique. What do you consider your weaknesses to be. Write down any queries to ask your swimming instructor.

DON'T – Forget to keep hydrated. You are exercising so you can still dehydrate, even though you are surrounded by water!

## REWARD

**Have a takeaway of your choice to celebrate getting this far.**

regular part of your life. It's all to do with the physical exertion stimulating and releasing chemicals in your brain so that you feel happier. So three cheers for those good old 'happy' chemicals.

Other benefits are a bit more mundane, but nice nonetheless. Because swimming is such a good sport for building fitness *and* strength, even tasks like carrying the shopping bags in from the car, or walking to the train station in the morning, will no longer have you huffing and puffing.

But don't get carried away with this feeling and start setting all sorts of other targets. As we said at the start of this programme, you should not change too much at once. Keep focused on your end goal of a 400-metre swim, and other benefits (weight loss etc) will follow naturally.

When you set the goal to swim 400 metres a few weeks back, you unknowingly released your subconscious to attract those things needed to get there. So as you keep training you will find yourself gradually drawn to other strategies that help you, such as better technique and nutrition.

Now onto your target goal: you swimming 400 metres. There are still a few weeks to go, plenty of time to get those muscles ready, so if you haven't already done it, then now is the time to start thinking

# 5days

*Now you have started exercising you are well on your way to meeting guidelines set out by many government health experts – adults aged over 18 should exercise at moderate intensity for 30 minutes at least five days per week. The exercise does not need to be consecutive but should be in bouts of at least 10 minutes at a time. (10)*

"He who has health has hope; and he who has hope has everything."

**ARABIC PROVERB**

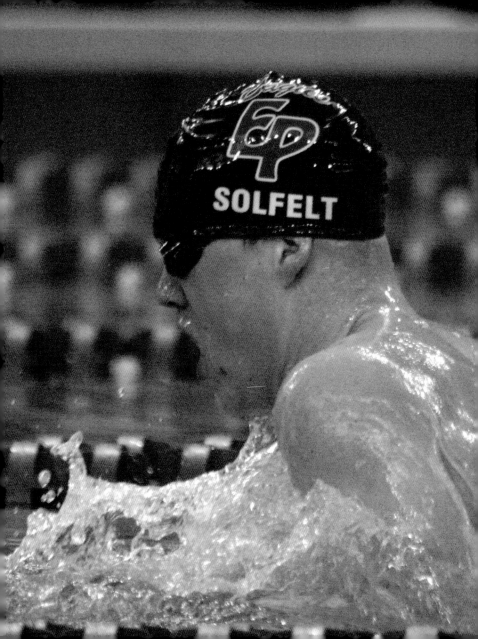

# Calories burnt in 30 mins

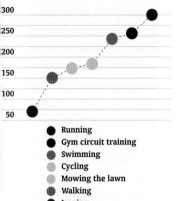

300
250
200
150
100
50

- ● Running
- ● Gym circuit training
- ● Swimming
- ● Cycling
- ● Mowing the lawn
- ● Walking
- ● Ironing

Different activities use up varying amounts of energy and it's worth noting that even some daily activities help keep you healthy.

The chart shows figures for a walking lawn mower, brisk walking at 6.5 kph (4 mph), moderate cycling at 19-22 kph (12-14 mph), swimming at a pace of 46 metres (50 yards) a minute, and running at 9.5 kph (6 mph). (11)

about where you will complete your challenge. Unlike for a sport such as running, where you'll find a wide choice of races every week, there are very few similar such organized races for casual swimmers. One option is to keep your eyes open for charity races, or sponsored swims put together by a school or by other community organizations.

However, it is more likely that you are going to have to plan your own 'race' on your challenge day. You can, of course, make it a solo event and head off to your local pool (we are assuming here, that not many of you have an idyllic lake at the bottom of your garden). But come on, you have trained hard for this, so why not grab your partner, family or friends (or all of them) and make a great day of it. Making an 'event' of it like this will also give you an added spur in the coming weeks.

Remember to choose a time when the pool is quiet so you won't be disturbed by too many other people splashing around. We've set your challenge day for either Saturday or Sunday (see page 131) to give you a bit of flexibility on this. Many pools have set times when they put out lane markers to separate lanes for people who want to do lengths. But if these times don't coincide with your planned challenge date then try to have a friendly word with the pool manager. Then come 'race day' it's down to you, your energy and a stopwatch.

"A wise man would consider that health is the greatest of human blessings."

**HIPPOCRATES**

# that's it!

## Week six completed

 You can enjoy all the positive feelings of exercising knowing there is more to come.

 You are not trying to change everything in your life at once. Concentrating on the programme is enough for now.

 You know that when you set your goal to swim 400 metres you released your subconscious to work towards that goal. The more you keep training, the more you will be drawn to things that will help you reach that goal.

 You have thought about where you will complete your challenge. Finalizing the details in your mind will bring the day more clearly into focus.

Your notes at the
end of the week

# week seven

**Keep it going**

**The end is in sight, but there is nothing to worry about if you've followed the programme…**

When a target is a long way off (as it was when you started this 400-metre swim programme) there is usually little to worry about. "There's plenty of time, so it'll be easy to sort things out and get to the end successfully," goes the thinking. This is because the target doesn't feel real because the end seems so far away. Now you are well into the programme though, the end is in sight, and with this comes some worries.

You now find yourself counting off the days (not the weeks) to the end of the challenge, and maybe panicking that you are never going to make it. "I need more training," and "I need more time," could be your mantras right now. But this is the time when you should be congratulating yourself on how far you have come. If you have followed the training programme to date then you will be well set up to finish your 400-metre swim challenge successfully.

It's common to worry that you are not ready, but remind yourself you do not have to be ready *right*

## YOUR AIM THIS WEEK

Is keep your mind on the end goal and not worry that you need to do extra training.

Now the end is in sight it will be more real, but there is no need to panic. The programme has been guiding you carefully along the path to success and there's still plenty of time.

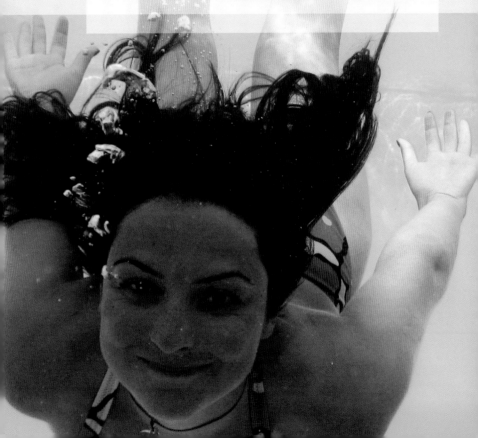

"You can never cross the ocean unless you have the courage to lose sight of the shore."

**CHRISTOPHER COLUMBUS**

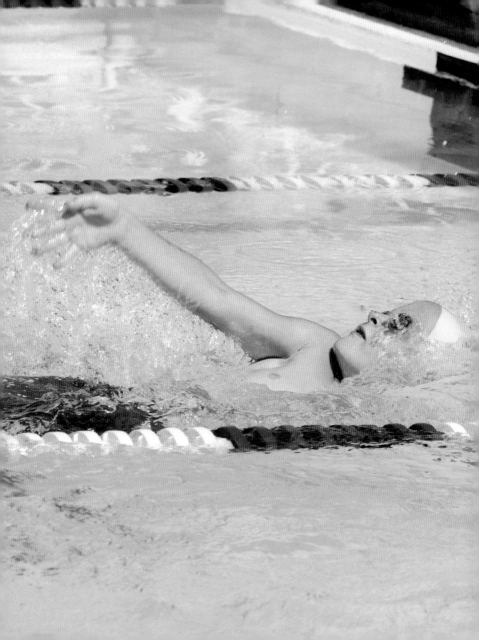

**YOUR DAILY NOTES**

| | | |
|---|---|---|
| **MON** | Rest. Resist the temptation to do too much. This week sees training increase, so you will need plenty of rest. | |
| **TUE** | Warm-up, then swim 100 metres (4 lengths). Rest for 5 minutes. Focus on technique and breathing. Repeat x 3. | |
| **WED** | Walk 10 mins briskly. Remember to apply the same principles of warming-up and cooling down to any exercise. | |
| **THU** | Warm-up, then swim 50 metres (2 lengths). Rest for 10 secs. Focus on technique and breathing. Repeat x 6. | |
| **FRI** | Walk 14 mins slowly. | |
| **SAT** | Rest. | |
| **SUN** | Warm-up, then swim 200 metres (8 lengths). Rest for 5 mins, then cool down. Focus on a relaxed stroke and good breathing. | |

## THIS WEEK

 DO – Review your progress so far. If you feel the programme is too much at this point, cut some of the sessions down. Schedule an extra day's rest if you feel you need it.

 CONSIDER – Joining a swimming club. You may benefit from the extra instruction and the support of like-minded members who may have similar goals.

DON'T – Get involved in racing other swimmers in the pool. Stick to your programme and look for small but lasting improvements.

## REWARD

A big bar
of chocolate
all to yourself!

*now*. Even though the end is in sight, and therefore more real, there is still plenty of time left in this programme, so trust in the training you have done and keep working hard. The programme has been devised so you make steady progress toward the final day of the challenge. Keep reminding yourself of that and stick with it.

Focus on your positive days (remind yourself what you did on those days and repeat the actions), and worry less about the bad days. You have to accept there are some bad training days, but allocate these to your short-term memory and keep the good days in your long-term memory.

You can help yourself with this by reviewing the notes you have written after each session and at the end the week. Use the good stuff like, "I'm loving this training because it makes me feel so energized," to motivate yourself. And laugh at the early struggles like, "I'm huffing and puffing like a steam train every time I get out of the pool". Those days are now behind you, but you can measure you progress just by reading those notes.

Do you enjoy raising money for charity? There is nothing like a sporting challenge to inspire people, so consider using your 400-metre swim challenge to help raise money for a good cause. Choose a charity that is close to your heart and send off an

**7,8,9**

*Most of us grow up being told that we need a 'good eight hours sleep' every night. Experts recommend seven to nine hours sleep a night for an adult – only you will know what is right for you. Try to get into a regular sleep pattern instead of trying to 'catch up' on the weekends as this re-sets your sleep cycle. (12)*

"The true reward for a thing well done is to have been the one who did it."

**ANON**

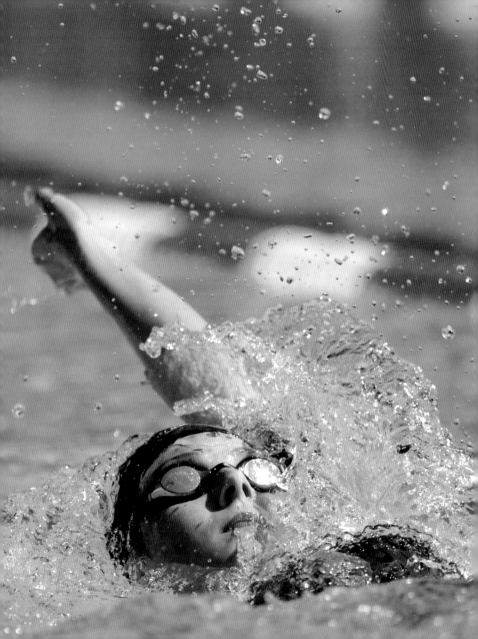

## Health benefits of fitness

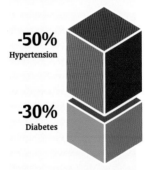

**-50%**
**Hypertension**

**-30%**
**Diabetes**

Exercising regularly reduces your risk of contracting many chronic diseases. These include Hypertension (50%), Ischaemic heart disease (40%), breast cancer (27%), a stroke (27%). (13)

e-mail explaining your plans. Most charities will have fundraising kits, including posters, collection boxes, and sponsorship forms they will send you. If not then ask for a letter from them confirming you are doing your swim challenge to raise money for them and set up your own forms to help raise some money. Supporting a charity also means you are firming up your commitment for your challenge and will be less likely to back out (not that you are thinking of that anyway, of course).

Are you training with someone else? A training buddy is great to keep you going but a little unhealthy competition can creep in sometimes. It's natural that one of you will be getting fitter quicker than the other as this programme progresses but try to avoid comparisons. You should not be competing with each other. You should be helping each other get to the end goal of your 400-metre swims.

There's nothing wrong with a little bit of fun competition with a friend to help push each other a little harder in training, but remember you started this challenge for yourself. If your buddy seems to be doing better than you then just keep focused on your own progress. If the golden swimming cap is on the other head, and you are the one doing better, then don't gloat, just keep encouraging your buddy. The goal has always been for you to complete a 400-metre swim.

"If you want to learn to swim jump into the water. On dry land no frame of mind is ever going to help you."

**BRUCE LEE**

# that's it!

## Week seven completed

 You know you should not be doing extra training even if you are getting worried about your progress. Trust in the programme and keep working hard.

 You have reviewed your notes and drawn inspiration from the progress you have made already.

 You are not competing with other people, especially if you have a training buddy. This challenge is all about you so the only progress you need to be concerned with is your own

 You have passed the halfway mark in your swimming programme. Give yourself a pat on the back!

Your notes at the end of the week

# week eight

## Recommit to your swim challenge

**Look ahead to the finish with confidence and recommit to the 400-metre challenge...**

Hands up if you didn't like that bit at the beginning of the programme when you had to tell five people about your plan to swim 400 metres? Oh dear, did you put up your hand? Well, now you are entering the home straight (that went quick didn't it?) it's time to repeat the exercise. Your recommitment to the challenge is an important part of the process so no skipping it.

It should certainly be easier this time around, even if you really are squeamish about being in the spotlight. Some friends and colleagues have undoubtedly been following your swimming progress and asking for updates anyway, so it won't be a surprise to them, and they will be more receptive to what you have to say.

As with the first time you did it, this doesn't have to be a dramatic, 'shout it from the rooftops' exercise. Far from it. In fact the whole point of doing this again is so you hear it yourself. So keep it casual. There will

### YOUR AIM THIS WEEK

Is to repeat the visualization exercise from week one – this time with more details added in.

Your mind is a powerful tool, and will work together with your body in getting you to end of your swim successfully. Run through this mind exercise as many times as you can as the swim approaches.

"The only prudence
in life is concentration."

**RALPH WALDO EMERSON**

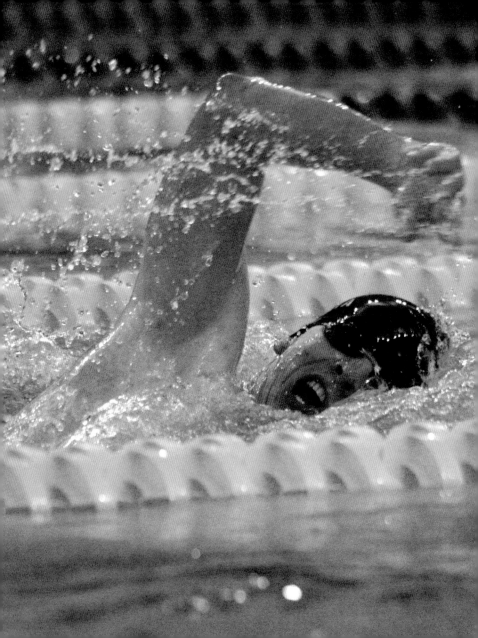

# WEEK EIGHT: YOUR TRAINING PROGRAMME AND DIARY

| | | YOUR DAILY NOTES |
|---|---|---|
| **MON** | Rest. | |
| **TUE** | Swimming lesson with qualified instructor. | |
| **WED** | Walk 10 mins briskly. | |
| **THU** | Warm-up, then swim 50 metres (2 lengths). Rest for 15 secs. Focus on technique and breathing. Repeat x 6. | |
| **FRI** | Walk 14 mins slowly. | |
| **SAT** | Rest. | |
| **SUN** | Warm-up, then swim 250 metres (10 lengths). Rest for 5 mins, then cool down. Focus on a relaxed stroke and good breathing. | |

## THIS WEEK

 DO – Ensure that you eat a snack within 30 minutes of exercise as this is the optimum window for replenishing lost energy stores.

CONSIDER – Changing your posture, particularly the way you sit. Look to support your back and avoid slouching, as this puts pressure on the spine.

DON'T – Get despondent if you have to miss the odd session. Accept that you may have other commitments, then get back to your programme as soon as you can.

## REWARD

Treat yourself to a night out at the cinema and switch off completely.

always be an opportunity to drop a positive comment into a conversation with a friend. "Oh I meant to say, I'm over halfway in the swimming programme I told you about last time we met. I'm determined to finish it." It's as simple as that.

If you did decide to complete your swim for a charity this might also be a good time to put your plans into action. Passing a sponsorship form around at work, or sending out an e-mail to friends, are other ways to reconfirm your commitment. A popular way to do this is to register your, and the charity's details, with an online fundraising site so people are able to make their donations electronically.

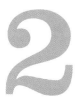

Another important part of your recommitment to your swim challenge is to repeat the visualization exercise – except this time you will be adding in more details. Now, you may be asking why there is a need to commit again? After all, you may be progressing swimmingly (sorry). But, unbelievably, some people do still drop out of fitness programmes, even at this stage.

Your mind is like your body when it comes to fitness. Just as you wouldn't expect your body to become fit after one training session, so it is with your mind. Keep working your mind with this visualization as often as you can in the coming weeks. Professional athletes spend a long time getting their minds ready

*Sports drinks contain two important ingredients – electrolytes (they help your muscles and heart function) and carbohydrates. You can lose electrolytes through very long workouts and the carbohydrates may help provide extra energy. Try sports drinks to see if they are for you, although water will always be important for most active people. (14)*

"Focus on the journey, not the destination. Joy is found not in finishing an activity but in doing it."

**GREG ANDERSON**

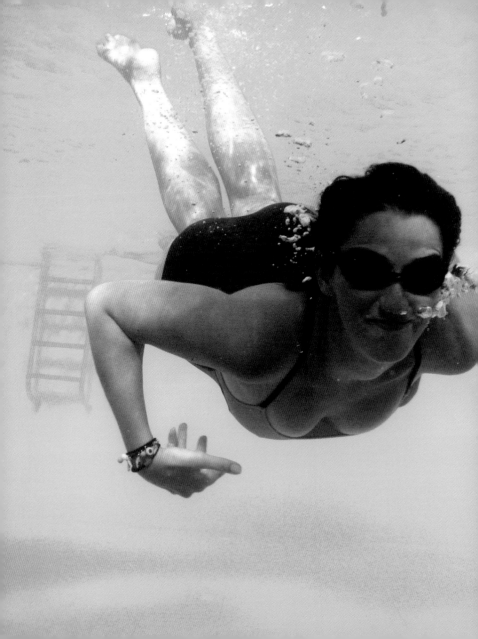

for their challenges, because they know the mind and body work together. Work on both and you will benefit from the power of the two working together.

Find somewhere quiet, where you won't be disturbed, and don't be afraid to close your eyes if it helps you to focus. Then start to fill in the details of your 400-metre swim. Picture yourself in the morning as you get ready to head off to the pool. 'See' yourself checking everything you have packed in your kit bag in preparation for the swim – your costume, your goggles, your towel, and so on. Then 'listen' to your favourite music as you head off to the pool.

## Calories in alcohol

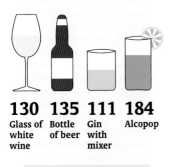

**130** Glass of white wine

**135** Bottle of beer

**111** Gin with mixer

**184** Alcopop

On a big night out it's easy to clock up the calories. The graphic shows figures for a 330 ml (11 fl oz) bottle of Stella Artois (4.8% abv), 175 ml (6 fl oz) glass of Jacob's Creek Chardonnay (13% abv), 25 ml (0.8 fl oz) of Bombay Sapphire (40% abv) and mixer, 275 ml (9 fl oz) WKD alcopop. (15)

Next, 'feel' the warmth of the air in the leisure centre as you get changed, and the heat of the water as you take your pre-swim shower. Take in all the sights and smells of the pool as you get ready, then 'feel' the water as you push away with your first stroke. Picture yourself swimming strongly and confidently as you count off the laps. You are now on the last couple of laps and the finish is in sight. Finally, imagine your feelings as you glide in to touch the side of the pool at the end of your 400 metres, then join your partner or friend to celebrate.

This is known as your 'future memory', something you have 'remembered', but which hasn't happened yet. It is a powerful tool to use and yet it takes just a few minutes.

"Talk doesn't
cook rice."

**CHINESE PROVERB**

# that's it!

## Week eight completed

 You are now well into the second half of this 12-week programme and still improving.

 You have told friends and family about your challenge again as a way of recommitting to it. If you are swimming for a charity then you have sent out details of how people can support you.

 You know your mind and body will work together towards achieving the goal you set at the beginning. Your mind is powerful so keep it positive.

 You have pictured your challenge day and filled in as many of the details as possible in your mind.

Your notes at the end of the week

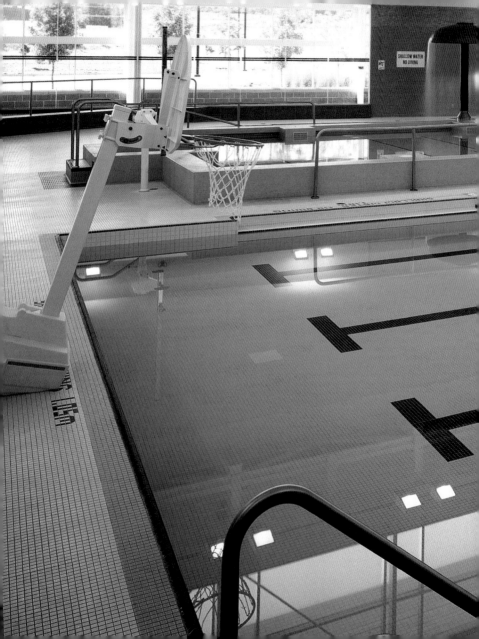

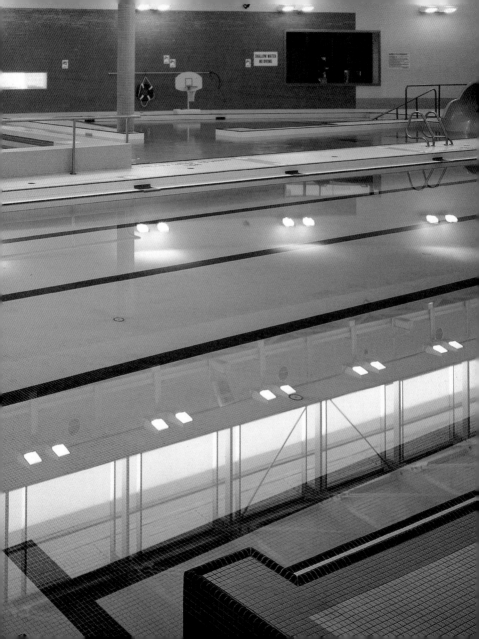

# week nine

## Taking care of the details

**It's time to refine your swimming technique…**

The best way to get better at something is to do it. This is why earlier in the programme we urged you to swim, swim and swim some more. At the start it was simply about getting back in the water and shaking off that swimming rustiness. Then it was about slowly building up your fitness and learning to enjoy exercising again. Now is a good time for you to review your technique in a bit more detail. A good technique leads to smoother swimming, meaning you will travel further in the water with less effort. Now that can't be bad can it?

Earlier in the book we recommended you use the breaststroke as you train towards your end goal. Although clearly not the fastest stroke, it is probably the most comfortable for the majority of people who have been away from swimming for a lengthy period. To make it more efficient concentrate getting your arms and legs to work together. It's easy if you have strong legs to let them dominate the movement of the upper body and vice versa, so always work on getting the correct timing between

**YOUR AIM THIS WEEK**

Is to take a bit of time to look closer at your swimming stroke.

Improving simple things such as how to get your arms and legs working together can dramatically improve your performance in the water. Small changes can mean faster swimming for less effort.

"If ifs were gifts
every day would
be Christmas."

**CHARLES BARKLEY**

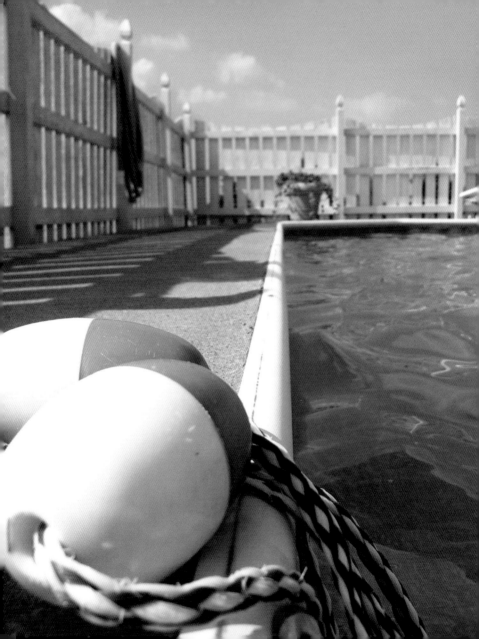

# **WEEK NINE:** YOUR TRAINING PROGRAMME AND DIARY

| | |
|---|---|
| **MON** | Rest. |
| **TUE** | Warm-up, then swim 100 metres (4 lengths). Rest for 20 seconds. Focus on technique and breathing. Repeat x 2. |
| **WED** | Walk 8 mins briskly. |
| **THU** | Warm-up, then swim 50 metres (2 lengths). Rest for 10 secs. Focus on technique and breathing. Repeat x 3. |
| **FRI** | Walk 10 mins slowly. |
| **SAT** | Rest. |
| **SUN** | Warm-up, then swim 200 metres (8 lengths). Rest for 5 mins, then cool down. Focus on a relaxed stroke and good breathing. |

## THIS WEEK

DO – Maintain a healthy dietary ratio of 50 per cent carbohydrates, 30 per cent protein and 20 per cent fats.

CONSIDER – Watching less TV. Read a book, or practise meditation, anything that relaxes rather than stimulates the mind.

DON'T – Try to be in two places at once like most people. Slow down! Focus on whatever task you happen to be doing and do it well.

## REWARD

A giant milk-shake full of goodness.

these two components to get the maximum benefit from each stroke.

Keep your body as flat as possible in the water and don't let your hips and legs 'sink and drag', although accept that as you lift your head to take a breath your body position will shift a bit. Avoid looking up, which will strain your neck, and instead keep your eyes looking down and forwards. This will also help you avoid your legs 'sinking and dragging', which effectively causes resistance and will slow you down, making your whole swim harder tougher.

On each stroke, stretch out as if you are trying to reach something in front of you, and use the palms of your hands like flippers to really push the water away, then turn them down and inwards as they come back through the stroke. Make sure you bring your feet up towards your backside and not underneath your body. Again, this is important, as pulling your feet up underneath your body will cause resistance and slow you down. Don't be afraid to really push your legs for extra propulsion rather than just going through the motions, but avoid breaking the water as this will reduce the power that is generated from your legs.

Breathe as you start to pull into each stroke, and work on fine-tuning your timing so you move from your body being fully stretched out to coiled like a frog ready for the pull of the next stroke. If you lose

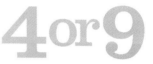

*Sugars and starches (carbohydrates) found in foods such as pasta, bread, cereal, fruit and vegetables have four calories per gram (0.14 oz) while fat is more than double at nine calories per gram (0.32 oz). Worth knowing when you're trying to get fit and healthy don't you reckon?* (16)

"You can do what you have to do, and sometimes you can do it even better than you think you can."

**JIMMY CARTER**

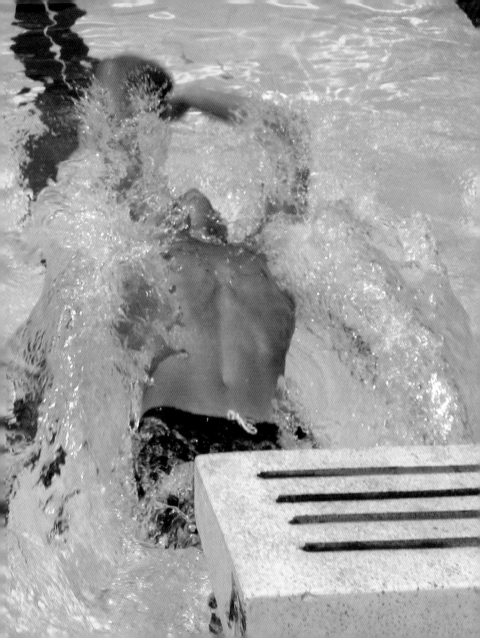

your rhythm, which is easy to do, especially when you get tired, just slow down to regain your composure and slowly get back into your stroke again.

If your preferred stroke is front crawl you will be getting a lot more bang for your bucks, especially if you can maintain your technique, but this is going to be very difficult over the full 400 metres. To be efficient you need to breath only on every second stroke at least, and a lack of air can make it difficult it you are an inexperienced swimmer or just getting back into the sport after a break. However, you may decide to alternate strokes and use front crawl for certain periods.

Concentrate on keeping your body in a streamlined position, and when breathing keep your head movement smooth to maintain this efficient position, rather than 'snatching' it sideways as you gulp for air. As one arm enters the water, the other one should be pulling round through the water to continue the circular movement. Turning your hips and shoulders will assist in this movement. Meanwhile, your legs should be kicking away at a steady pace and there should be minimal knee flexion.

If you use backstroke, keep your eyes facing to the ceiling and your ears at the surface. Keep your head still and turn your shoulders and hips, which will allow your arms to come over for each stroke. Use an alternating leg kick and try to keep your chest and shoulders high in the water.

## A balanced diet

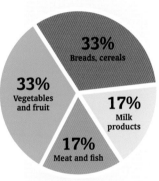

**33%**
Breads, cereals

**33%**
Vegetables and fruit

**17%**
Milk products

**17%**
Meat and fish

Try to maintain a balanced diet of the 'basic four food groups' in the proportions shown in the chart above and to eat from all of them every day. Also limit the amount of fats you include in your diet. (17)

"If you refuse to accept anything but the best, you very often get it."

**WILLIAM SOMERSET MAUGHAM**

# that's it!

## Week nine completed

 You have reminded yourself that the best way to get better at something is to do it. So keep swimming, and swimming more.

 You know that on all swimming strokes keeping a streamlined body is everything. Concentrate on keeping your body high in the water and keeping movements smooth.

 You know in breaststroke you should use your palms like flippers to push away the water, and to pull your feet towards your backside and not let them fall underneath you.

 You know with front crawl that as one arm enters the water the other should already be pulling through the water so it is ready for the next stroke.

**Your notes at the end of the week**

# week ten

## Keep your mind on track

**You're feeling strong, but don't get over-confident. There is still some work to do...**

This swimming is becoming a doddle isn't it? A few weeks ago you were worried about completing a couple of lengths without stopping, now here you are in Week 10, poised for success. Just to put it into perspective: in Week 1 the 'long swim' on Sunday was just two lengths, while this week the Sunday swim is 12 lengths – three-quarters of the way towards your challenge target.

This is the last week of heavy work; after this the workload will decrease to ensure you remain fresh for your challenge day. However, don't think you need to power your way through this week to prove something. Keep your swims smooth and easy and use the last planned session with your swimming instructor to iron out any last-minute worries.

A few weeks ago we urged you to avoid the temptation to do more training than is set out for you in the programme even if you felt you had not done enough. This is the, "I need to squeeze in a

### YOUR AIM THIS WEEK

Is to guard against over-confidence as you approach the home straight on this challenge.

Over-confidence can mean you push yourself too hard in training and ruin all your hard work. Trust the programme and it will guide you to end successfully.

"Pleasure and action make the hours seem short."

**WILLIAM SHAKESPEARE**

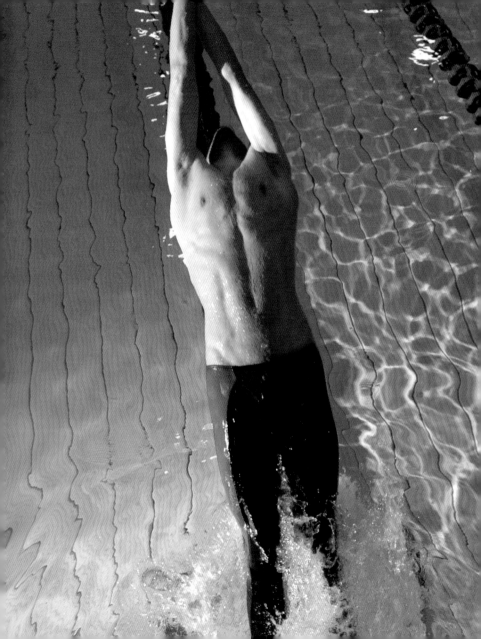

**YOUR DAILY NOTES**

| | |
|---|---|
| **MON** | Rest. |
| **TUE** | Swimming lesson with qualified instructor. |
| **WED** | Walk 8 mins briskly. |
| **THU** | Warm-up, then swim 50 metres (2 lengths). Rest for 10 secs. Focus on technique and breathing. Repeat x 6. |
| **FRI** | Walk 12 mins slowly. |
| **SAT** | Rest. |
| **SUN** | Warm-up, then swim 300 metres (12 lengths). Rest for 5 mins, then cool down. Focus on a relaxed stroke and good breathing. |

## THIS WEEK

DO – Share your progress with friends and family. Use your example to inspire others as well as yourself.

CONSIDER – Keeping a more detailed journal of your training to record how the programme is going.

DON'T – Lose sight of your target. Reaffirm your commitment every now and then to help you stay focused.

## REWARD

Treat yourself to a spa and sauna.

few more swims just to make sure I get to the finish successfully," type of approach.

Now we need to warn against something just as damaging – over-confidence. This is the, "I can do anything, I am super strong," style of thinking. Both will result in making you tired and less likely to finish the 400-metre swim come challenge day. Don't ruin all your hard work at this late stage by getting too big for your swimming goggles.

What happens with over-confidence is this… You head off with your training buddy for a session (let's say Thursday's swim 50 metres, rest for 10 seconds, repeat six times session). You warm-up together, then complete the first 50 metres in a nice, steady pace. This carries on until there are only a couple of repeats left. Your buddy is puffing but you think you are a Superhero from a comic book (choose your favourite). You even have the bright Lycra outfit.

So you head into your metaphorical telephone booth, then announce to your buddy you are really going push yourself on these last couple of repeats because you are feeling strong. You zip off like Madman (not a well-known Superhero, but the star of this show), leaving your training partner in your wake. But he has more sense than you and sticks to the normal training pace. You finish way ahead and sit on the side of the pool (all smug) as your buddy comes in. But while he

**17-19**

Researchers in Australia and New Zealand found that people who drove after being awake for 17-19 hours performed worse than those who had a blood-alcohol level of 0.5 per cent – the legal limit for drivers in Australia and many European countries. It's not difficult to see that sleep is important for anyone who wants to focus on his/her health and fitness. (18)

"I may not be there yet but I am closer than I was yesterday."

ANON

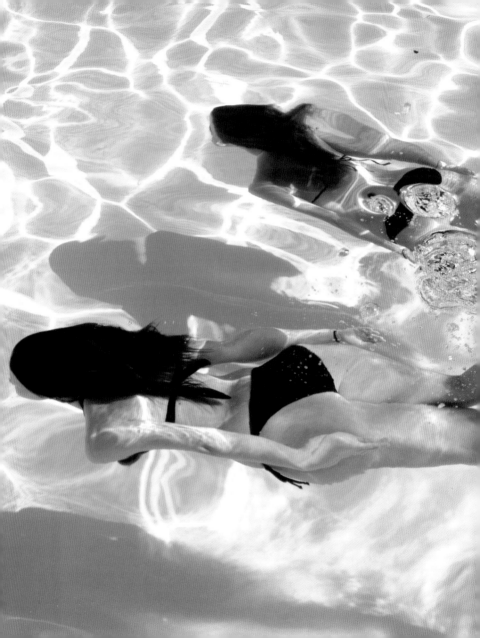

## The human body

**60%**
**Water**

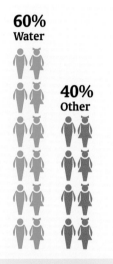

**40%**
**Other**

Around 55-60 per cent of your body is made up of water. Your brain is 70 per cent water, blood 83 per cent water and lungs nearly 90 per cent. Make sure you keep yourself topped up by drinking plenty of water throughout the day. (19)

has added another important building block to his training, you have knocked a few of your own down by draining your energy. Come race day, guess which one of you finishes strongly and confidently, and who battles the whole way (or worse still, may even fail to finish altogether)? Don't let over-confidence get the better of you.

Are you aiming for a particular time during your race? We have avoided discussion of this because the programme's aim is to get you to the end of the 400-metre swim successfully. However, it is inevitable that as you got stronger during the programme you may have set a specific time target. Good luck if you do have a target, but don't let it interfere with the completion of your swim as with the story above. Rather, keep focused on the end goal – the performance – and a desired outcome of a particular time should follow.

Now, how about some good news? Moderate exercise means you strengthen your immune system, so your chance of catching a cold is lower than it was before you started exercising. But it can still happen, and it really is frustrating just as you are wrapping up a fitness programme. Do everything you would normally to avoid picking up a bug (such as keeping warm, washing your hands regularly, and so on). However, if you do get sick do not keep training, and consult a doctor.

"I am building a
fire, and everyday
I train, I add
more fuel. At
just the right
moment, I light
the match."

**MIA HAMM**

# that's it!

## Week ten completed

 You are now wondering why you didn't start swimming earlier, because it is becoming second nature to you.

 You have had your last planned session with your swimming instructor. Use the session to talk through any last-minute worries about your technique or your motivational levels. Chat through how you can get these right for your challenge day.

 You are warding off the dreaded danger of over-confidence. You are not a Superhero, even with the Lycra outfit, so keep things easy in your training.

You know you are less likely to pick up a bug than when you started this programme, because exercise boosts your immune system. However, if you do get sick, consult a doctor.

**Your notes at the end of the week**

**Not long now**

**Concentrate on the challenge and avoid taking on new projects…**

Do you have a long list of projects you want to do? You know the sort of things – put up new shelves in the study, fix the shed roof, or clean out the boxes in the garage.

The reason most of us have a long list is we think of new things to add to it (or our partner does), faster than we tick off the ones already on it. But despite this, you are probably happy to have your list tucked away in the back of your mind. Yes, sometimes it nags away at you, and hey, surprise surprise, occasionally you get round to doing one of the jobs. But by and large you can live happily side by side with your mostly undone list.

It's understandable that you look at the list when you are bored (and you really would have to be incredibly bored to clean out the boxes in the garage). But why is it you also dig out the list when you actually have something important to do? The reason is, quite simply, to try to distract yourself.

**YOUR AIM THIS WEEK**

Is to keep you mind on your swimming challenge and avoid taking on new projects to distract you from your nerves.

You can't control everything in your life – you will always have work, family and social responsibilities – so concentrate on the things you can control.

"The secret
of success is
constancy
of purpose."

**BENJAMIN DISRAELI**

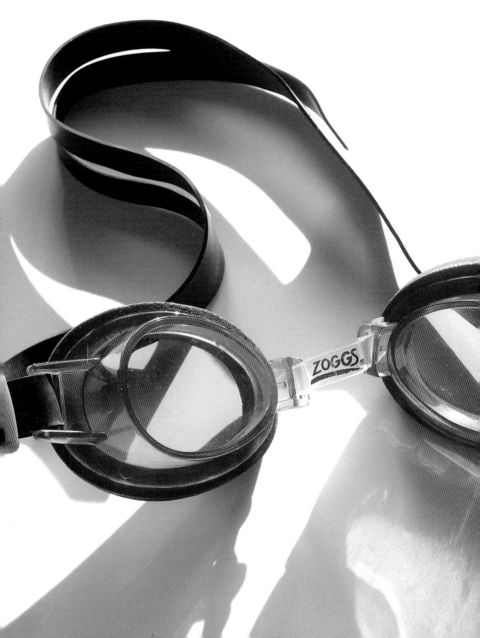

**YOUR DAILY NOTES**

| | |
|---|---|
| **MON** | Rest. From now on, your overall training begins to decrease in order to conserve energy for your goal. |
| **TUE** | Warm-up, then swim 100 metres (4 lengths). Rest for 20 secs. Focus on technique and breathing. Repeat x 3. |
| **WED** | Walk 8 minutes briskly. |
| **THU** | Warm-up, then swim 200 metres (8 lengths). Rest for 20 secs. Focus on technique and breathing. Repeat x 2. |
| **FRI** | Walk 12 mins slowly. |
| **SAT** | Rest. |
| **SUN** | Warm-up, then swim 300 metres (12 lengths). Rest for 5 mins, then cool down. Focus on a relaxed stroke and good posture. |

## THIS WEEK

 DO – Take time out whenever you can and remind yourself that rest is an integral part of any exercise programme.

CONSIDER – Walking on short journeys, as an alternative to taking the car.

 DON'T – Forget to warm-up and cool down at each session. Failure to do so can effect your overall performance and lead to injury.

## REWARD

A nice new bag for your swimming equipment.

The minute something becomes important you stand to lose something if you fail, so to distract yourself from thoughts of failure you look at doing something mundane.

Avoid taking on new projects at this stage, even as the excitement mounts. If a box of books has already been waiting in the corner for months for the new shelves to go up in the study, will another couple more weeks really hurt? Your 400-metre swim challenge is now only a couple of weeks away and you need to concentrate fully on this both mentally and physically. So tuck that list back into the recesses of your mind, where it belongs for now.

**36°C**

If you do need to distract yourself, choose something relaxing like lounging in front of an-easy-to-watch film, reading a book or flicking through a magazine.

Avoiding projects like these is one of the few things you can control. But there are, of course, many things you cannot control. Unlike a professional athlete, who would live, breathe and sleep for the end goal, you have a life to lead. There are always work colleagues, children, your partner, parents, and friends, who demand a bit of your time.

> *Be particularly careful when exercising in hot weather. Once the temperature rises to 36°C (97°F) it is recommended you cancel your session or postpone it to a cooler part of the day as the heat will put a lot of stress on your body. [20]*

Time pressures from all sides were probably one of the main reasons you ended up in your armchair with a large pizza every night in the first place. But, over

"Success doesn't come to you... you go to it."

MARVA COLLINS

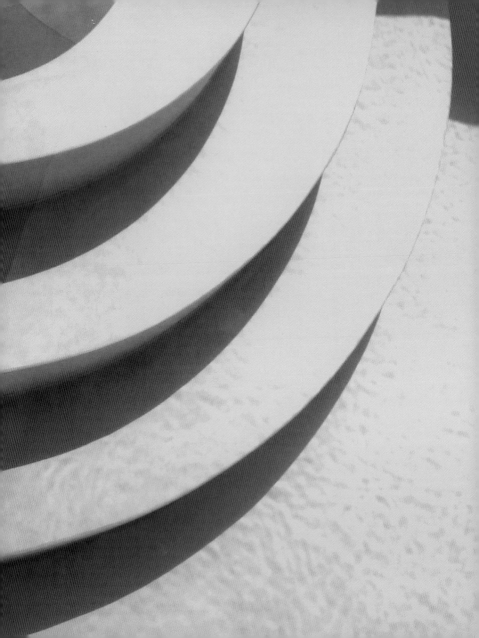

## A balanced meal

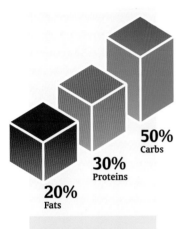

**50%**
Carbs

**30%**
Proteins

**20%**
Fats

Try to balance all food elements with every meal you eat in line with the figures shown in the chart above.

Carbohydrates include rice, bread, fruits and vegetables, proteins come from meat, fish, milk products and eggs, while nuts, avocados, green olives, fish oil and olive oil are a good source of fats. (21)

the last few weeks, you have proved you are able to make time for your swimming and still meet all those demands. Keep what you do to a minimum in the next couple of weeks so you stay fresh mentally and physically. Concentrate on the things you can control.

Things to concentrate on at this stage are eating and sleeping well, and drinking plenty of water. It's also a good idea to ease up on the alcohol. This is not the part where we expect you to transform your eating habits (this is not the time for your digestive system to be messed with), but there are few basics you should try to stick to.

Firstly breakfast. All together now, what is breakfast? Let's hear it… That's right, "Breakfast is the most *important* meal of the day!" We've heard it so many times before but it's true. Try to have something simple like yoghurt, porridge, muesli, or a sandwich with some light cream cheese. Just have something. For the day get a couple of healthy snacks ready – a piece of fruit or some nuts – for when you are feeling hungry between meals.

When it comes to liquid, you should already be in the habit of drinking water during the day. Remember to top up regularly. Also ease up on the alcohol as it will dehydrate you. This doesn't mean you have to lock up the drinks cupboard, but a week of heavy nights right now is not going to do you much good.

"In each of us are places where we have never gone. Only by pressing the limits do you ever find them."

**JOYCE BROTHERS**

# that's it!

## Week eleven completed

 You know you can't control everything – you will always have work and family commitments – so you will concentrate on the things you can control.

 You know one of the things you can control is that list of 'things to do' you have tucked away in your mind. This is not the time to be tackling that list.

 You are keeping hydrated during the day by drinking lots of water and getting a good sleep every night.

 You know alcohol will dehydrate you and this will affect your performance. A glass of wine won't hurt but don't overdo it.

Your notes at the
end of the week

# week twelve

**All your hard work gets put into practice this week. Go for it…**

This is the moment of truth then. Or at least the week of truth. Are you ready? Are you raring to go? Of course you are. You've done the hard work, followed the training programme, now you can enjoy a nice easy week before your 400-metre swim

Sessions are easier this week (just a couple of 20-minute swims plus a couple of short walks) so enjoy them, making sure to keep nice and loose. Depending on whether you have chosen Saturday or Sunday for your challenge day, you will have one or two days of rest leading up to it. Treat these rest days with respect, as they are important for your body, and will ensure that you are fresh come the day of the swim. However, a little bit of gentle stretching is recommended on these days so your muscles don't tighten up.

It is important you are prepared and get everything ready for your day in advance. Go through the checklist below and get you bag ready early.

### YOUR AIM THIS WEEK

Is to enjoy the last week, then tackle your challenge successfully.

You have spent weeks training for this swim so you should be in shape to complete it without problems. Head off with the confidence that you can do it.

"People with goals will succeed because they know where there are going."

**EARL NIGHTINGALE**

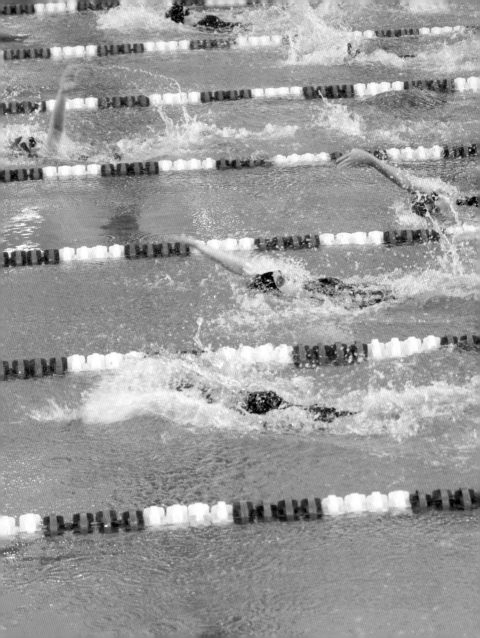

# **WEEK TWELVE:** YOUR TRAINING PROGRAMME AND DIARY

| | | |
|---|---|---|
| **MON** | Rest. This is it! Your big week has arrived, so take it easy. | |
| **TUE** | Warm-up, then swim 50 metres (2 lengths). Rest for 10 seconds. Focus on your technique and breathing. Repeat x 4. | |
| **WED** | Walk 5 mins briskly. | |
| **THU** | Warm-up, then swim 100 metres (4 lengths). Rest for 10 secs. Focus on technique and breathing. Repeat x 2. | |
| **FRI** | Walk 8 mins slowly. Or rest. | |
| **SAT** | Goal event! Swim 400 metres (16 lengths). Rest for 5 mins, then cool down. (Or rest day). Choose the day which is best for you to complete the challenge. | |
| **SUN** | Goal event! Swim 400 metres (16 lengths). Rest for 5 mins, then cool down. (Or rest day). Choose the day which is best for you to complete the challenge. | |

## THIS WEEK

 DO – Get plenty of sleep in the build-up to your target. Relax and put your feet up whenever you can.

CONSIDER – Setting future goals. Perhaps an increase in distance or an organized event like a charity swim or a race.

DON'T – Eat less than two hours before exercise. Stick to a healthy diet and your energy stores will be more than adequate.

## REWARD

Give yourself a pat on the back for achieving your goal!

## Checklist

- ☐ Swimming kit
- ☐ Swimming cap
- ☐ Goggles
- ☐ Money for locker
- ☐ Jacket or warm top
- ☐ Towel

- ☐ Water bottle or sports drink
- ☐ Energy bar
- ☐ Stopwatch
- ☐ Camera for souvenir photos afterwards!

You might find it difficult to sleep the night before the swim because of nerves, so try to get as much good sleep as you can this week. Have a decent dinner (but nothing too heavy) the night before your challenge and drink plenty of water to make sure you are well hydrated in the morning. If you have chosen an early start in the morning to avoid the crowds in the pool, then try to get to bed a bit earlier than usual.

In the morning, top up with water and make sure you eat something at least two hours before the start of your swim. Remember, you can't take on liquids during your swim, so it's important you are properly hydrated at the start. Stick to your usual breakfast and don't eat things your stomach is not used to.

If you've been lucky enough to have found a charity race or sponsored swim, then get to the start early so you can get your bearings, and make sure you stay warm on your way to the pool. Try to have

## 6-10

*If you need a performance boost in the day then a short sleep – or a power nap if you want to sound smart – of just six to 10 minutes could do the trick. If this sounds like something for you then keep the nap short and sharp so you avoid waking up feeling groggy. (22)*

"What counts is not necessarily the size of the dog in the fight – it's the size of the fight in the dog."

**DWIGHT EISENHOWER**

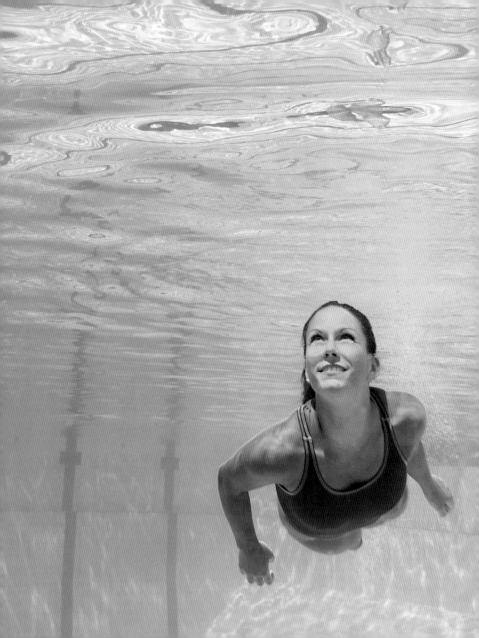

a shower before you get into the pool so you are warmed up and ready. Even if you have set up the swim challenge yourself, and there will be no official starting time, still try to stick to the schedule you have planned. Check with pool staff that the line markers are in place for you, if you have arranged that beforehand, and start at the time you have set for yourself. Take this seriously.

If you have had a training buddy during the programme then chat about your swim and remind each other of all the hard work you have put in, as this will help calm your nerves. Then soak up the goodwill of any friends or family that may have come along to encourage you on your 400-metre swim.

Don't get carried away and go charging off too fast at the start, even if you are feeling excited. This is an easy thing to do, so keep focused on getting a couple of easy lengths under your belt and establishing a nice, steady rhythm.

If the pool is busier than you'd hoped for, don't panic, just keeping moving steadily and try to keep your strokes as smooth as possible. Try to avoid weaving in and out of other people too much or you will be adding unwanted metres to your distance.

But finally, you are ready... now is the time to go out and enjoy your swim!

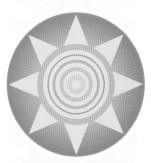

Have you ever noticed how refreshed and good you feel after exercising once the huffing and puffing has stopped?

Numerous studies have found there is a direct link between exercising and feeling happy and satisfied with your life. Getting a smile on your face – can there be a better reason for you to exercise? (23)

"I count him braver who overcomes his desires than him who conquers his enemies; for the hardest victory is over self."

**ARISTOTLE**

# that's it!

## Week twelve completed

 You have completed your target of a 400-metre swim in 12 weeks. Well done!

 You now have a full set of notes to remind yourself of what you have achieved over those 12 weeks.

 Your training has made you fitter and healthier and you have proved you can take on a challenge and tackle it successfully. Enjoy the feeling.

 You must be ready for a reward? We suggest a pat on the back, but we're sure you can think of something more fun!

Your notes at the
end of the week

# what now?

## You've done it! Now you can look ahead

**You've successfully completed your challenge.
What's next…**

The first thing you should do now you have finished
your 400-metre swimming challenge is to take a
short break. The break only has a be a few days,
whatever you feel is right, but try to stop training
for a short time.

This is to give your body a rest after the exertion of
the challenge, and also for psychological reasons.
Over the last few weeks you have been gearing up
mentally, as well as physically for this swim, and a
break will act as an punctuation point that signals
the end of the programme.

Don't let the break become too long or you may get
tempted to slip back into your old pizza-chomping
habits. Instead, use the few 'days off' to think back
over what you have already achieved and what, if
anything, you want to do next. You might, of course,
decide that's it and you don't want to carry on. But
that really would be a waste after you've spent so
much time and energy getting yourself back in shape.

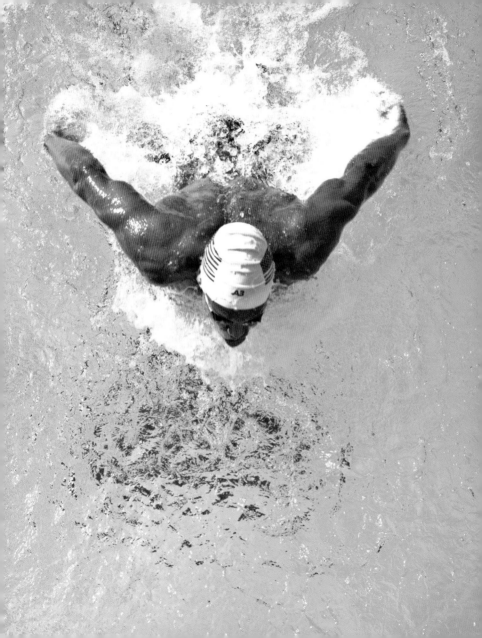

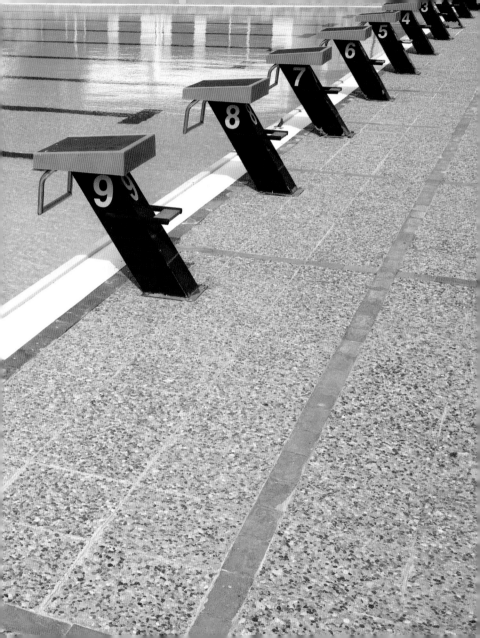

It's a lot easier to keep fit once you are there, than it is actually getting fit in the first place. You'll only have to think back to how tough the early training sessions were for evidence of this.

Maybe you are happy continuing as you are, with three swim sessions a week? This will certainly maintain the level of fitness you have reached over the past 12 weeks, but you also know this works for you from a time perspective. One thing you've probably discovered over the last few weeks is that you *can* find time to keep yourself fit and healthy and still meet all the other commitments you have in your life. You might find it helps if you set yourself another goal (how about 800 metres this time?). Having a goal gives you something to aim for and acts as a great motivator.

If you are feeling on top of the world after your achievements (and who can blame you?) then maybe you want to take your swimming to the next level. You could certainly book regular sessions with a swimming instructor to fine-tune your stroke technique (or learn another stroke). This may also be the time to join a swimming club and see just how far you can take it.

Remember, there's nothing to say you have to stick just to swimming to keep fit. Although swimming is great for an full body workout, you've also been doing a number of walks in the programme. These were included because it's important to work muscles in different ways, but also to avoid the monotony of doing the same thing all the time.

There are many different ways to keep fit, from gym sessions to dancing. Or try another sport like running or cycling. You could mix things up with a bit of swimming and a bit of running during the week. This approach of using different sports to keep fit certainly keeps your mind (as well as your body) fresh.

If you are really enthusiastic be careful you don't set yourself goals that are out of reach. There is no point trying to plan an hour's fitness training, six times a week, only to find other life pressures mean you can't keep it up. This leads to frustration and disappointment. If you want to do more training, then build up slowly, both for your body's sake and your mind's. Stretch yourself, by all means, but not to breaking point.

Whatever you decide to do going forward from your success with the 400-metre swim, remember to enjoy it. Keeping fit and healthy should not feel like a chore. When you were young you probably kept fit simply by running around and having fun with your friends. Try to keep that level of enthusiasm. A smile on your face as you exercise can go a long way. But most importantly, stick at it!

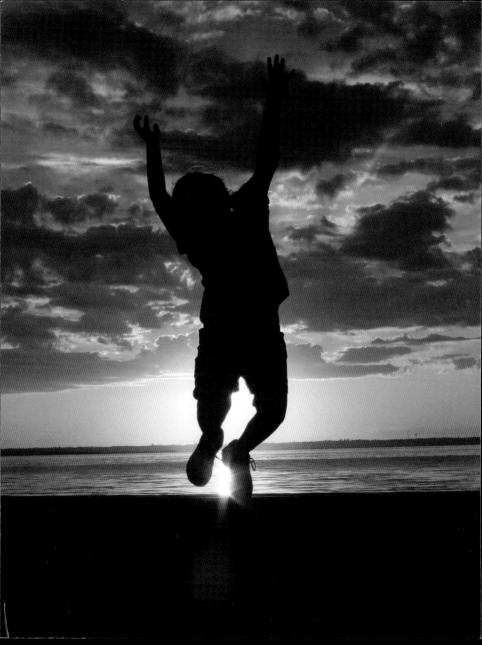

First published in 2013 by
New Holland Publishers (UK) Ltd
London • Cape Town • Sydney • Auckland
www.newhollandpublishers.com

A catalogue record for this book is available from the British Library.

ISBN 978 1 78009 235 5

This book has been produced for New Holland Publishers by
Chase My Snail Ltd
London • Cape Town
www.chasemysnail.com

Designer: Darren Exell
Photo Editor: Anthony Ernest
Proof reader: David Chapman, Tony Headley
Consultant sports psychologist: Russell Murphy
Production: Marion Storz

2 4 6 8 10 9 7 5 3 1

Printed and bound in China by Toppan Leefung Printing Ltd.